The Academic Health Center
and Health Care Reform

Conference Planning Committee

Ralph Snyderman, M.D., Chair
William G. Anlyan, M.D.
Arthur Garson, Jr., M.D., M.P.H.
J. Alexander McMahon, J.D.
Mark C. Rogers, M.D., M.B.A.
Vicki Y. Saito

The generous support of The Duke Endowment is gratefully acknowledged.

The Academic Health Center and Health Care Reform

Proceedings of The Duke Private Sector Conference 1994

Editors:

Ralph Snyderman, M.D.
Mark C. Rogers, M.D., M.B.A.
Vicki Y. Saito
Duke University Medical Center
Durham, North Carolina

Raven Press ✺ New York

Raven Press Ltd., 1185 Avenue of the Americas, New York, New York 10036

Made in the United States of America

Library of Congress Cataloging-in-Publication Data

Private Sector Conference (1994: Duke University)
    The academic health center and health care reform: proceedings of the Duke Private Sector Conference. 1994/editors, Ralph Snyderman, Mark C. Rogers, Vicki Y. Saito.
       p. cm.
    Includes bibliographical references.
    ISBN 0-7817-0326-3 (pbk.)
    1. Academic medical centers—Effect of managed care on—United States—Congresses. 2. Health care reform—United States—Congresses.
    I. Snyderman, Ralph. II. Rogers, Mark C. III. Saito, Vicki Y. IV. Title.
    [DNLM: 1. Academic Medical Centers—trends—United States—Congresses. 2. Health Care Reform—United States—Congresses.
WX 27 AA1 P96a   1995]
RA981.A2P67   1994
362.1'0937—dc20
DNLM/DLC
for Library of Congress   95-7174
                                                       CIP

9 8 7 6 5 4 3 2 1

Contents

xiii Overview
      Ralph Snyderman

xv Historical Perspective
      William G. Anlyan

Session I: The Health Care Environment

1 Introduction
      Ralph Snyderman

2 The Health System as a Mosaic of Cost Centers: The Economic
      Implications of Health Reform
      Uwe E. Reinhardt

11 Overview: The Evolution of the Academic Health Center in
      Health Care Reform
      Ralph Snyderman

19 All-Payer Funding Stream
      Brian Biles

21 Academic Health Centers Must Undergo Cultural Change
      Michael M. E. Johns

25 Price Will Determine Our Costs
      James E. Mulvihill

29 Free Associations
      Herbert Pardes

32 Responses
      Frank A. Sloan
      Louis W. Sullivan
      Robert Waller
      Virginia V. Weldon

37 General Discussion

Session II: Are the Missions of the AHC Relevant to Society?

45 Overview
      Arnold S. Relman

46 Looking to the Corporate Sector
   Thomas W. Langfitt

47 Competition in a Changing World
   Steven A. Schroeder

50 Toward Comprehensive Care
   Daniel C. Tosteson

52 Discussion

56 Responses
   Arthur Garson, Jr.
   William New, Jr.
   Robert G. Petersdorf

59 General Discussion

**Session III: How Will Health Care Delivery Systems
for the AHC Change in an Era of Reform?**

69 Overview
   Mark C. Rogers

72 The Need for Strategic Planning
   William N. Kelley

76 Partner Attributes
   James A. Lane

79 Philosophies of Survival
   Mitchell T. Rabkin

82 Swimming in the Same Sea
   David W. Singley, Jr.

85 Responses
   Joseph B. Martin
   Gary A. Mecklenburg
   Bruce J. Sams

90 General Discussion

Session IV: Conference Summary and Reflections

99 Dealing with the Inefficiencies
   William G. Anlyan

101   We Must Stand for Quality
         Roscoe R. Robinson

103   Government Control or Market Control?
         J. Alexander McMahon

105   General Discussion

Contributors

William G. Anlyan, M.D.

Dr. Anlyan is Chancellor Emeritus of Duke University and a trustee of The Duke Endowment. From 1964 to 1988, he was head of Duke University Medical Center.

Brian Biles, M.D., M.P.H.

Dr. Biles is Deputy Assistant Secretary for Public Health Policy.

Arthur Garson, Jr., M.D., M.P.H.

Dr. Garson is Associate Vice Chancellor for Health Affairs, the Geller Distinguished Professor of Pediatrics, Medicine and Public Policy, and Chief of Pediatric Cardiology at Duke University Medical Center.

Michael M. E. Johns, M.D.

Dr. Johns is Vice President for Medical Affairs and Dean of the School of Medicine at the Johns Hopkins University.

William N. Kelley, M.D.

Dr. Kelley is Executive Vice President of the University of Pennsylvania, where he also is Chief Executive Officer of the Medical Center and Health System, Dean of the School of Medicine and Robert G. Dunlop Professor of Medicine, Biochemistry and Biophysics.

James A. Lane, J.D.

Mr. Lane is a Senior Vice President of Kaiser Foundation Health Plan, Inc. and Kaiser Foundation Hospitals. He is the leader of Kaiser Permanente's Health Care Reform Team, which is charged with leading Kaiser Permanente's efforts to influence reform legislation.

Thomas W. Langfitt, M.D.

Dr. Langfitt is Chairman and Chief Executive Officer of The Glenmede Corporation and President and Chief Executive Officer of The Glenmede Trust Company, the parent organization to The Pew Charitable Trusts.

Joseph B. Martin, M.D., Ph.D.

Dr. Martin is Chancellor of the University of California, San Francisco. He was Dean of the UCSF School of Medicine from 1989 to 1993.

J. Alexander McMahon, J.D.

Mr. McMahon, who served 14 years as President of the American Hospital Association, is Executive-in-Residence with Duke University's Fuqua School of Business.

Gary A. Mecklenburg, M.B.A.

Mr. Mecklenburg is President and Chief Executive Officer of Northwestern Memorial Hospital and its parent organization, Northwestern Memorial Corporation.

James E. Mulvihill, D.M.D.

Since 1993, Dr. Mulvihill has been Senior Fellow in Health Policy at the Association of Academic Health Centers. Previously, he served as Senior Vice President for Health Policy of the Travelers Insurance Company and Chairman of The Travelers Health Company and Chairman of The Travelers Health Network.

William New, Jr., M.D., Ph.D.
Dr. New is Chairman and Chief Executive Officer of Natus Medical Incorporated. He also serves as Clinical Associate Professor at Stanford University Medical Center and Chairman of the Board of Visitors at Duke University Medical Center.

Herbert Pardes, M.D.
Dr. Pardes is Vice President for Health Sciences, Dean of the Faculty of Medicine and Chairman of the Department of Psychiatry at the College of Physicians and Surgeons, Columbia University.

Robert G. Petersdorf, M.D.
Dr. Petersdorf was President of the Association of American Medical Colleges for eight years when he retired on April 1, 1994. He is now President Emeritus of the AAMC and Professor of Medicine at the University of Washington.

Mitchell T. Rabkin, M.D.
Dr. Rabkin has been the President of Boston's Beth Israel Hospital for over 27 years.

Uwe E. Reinhardt, Ph.D.
Dr. Reinhardt, a native of Germany, has taught at Princeton University since 1968, rising through the ranks to his current position as James Madison Professor of Political Economy.

Arnold S. Relman, M.D.
Dr. Relman is Editor-in-Chief Emeritus of *The New England Journal of Medicine*, and Professor Emeritus of Medicine and Social Medicine at the Harvard Medical School.

Roscoe R. Robinson, M.D.
Dr. Robinson is Professor of Medicine and Vice Chancellor for Health Affairs at Vanderbilt University Medical Center.

Mark C. Rogers, M.D., M.B.A.
Dr. Rogers is Vice Chancellor for Health Systems at Duke University Medical Center and Chief Executive Officer of Duke University Hospital and the Health Network.

Bruce J. Sams, M.D.
For 30 years, Dr. Sams was a practicing internist in The Permanente Group (Kaiser Permanente, Northern California). Since his retirement from Kaiser Permanente in April 1993, he has been a private consultant in managed care.

Steven A. Schroeder, M.D.
Dr. Schroeder is President of the Robert Wood Johnson Foundation, the nation's largest health care philanthropy. He is also Clinical Professor of Medicine at The Robert Wood Johnson Medical School.

David W. Singley, Jr.
Mr. Singley has been President of Coastal Physician Services Group, Inc., a principal subsidiary of Coastal Healthcare Group, Inc., in Durham, N.C., since 1993. He became Chief Operating Officer of the company on January 1, 1994.

Frank A. Sloan, Ph.D.
Frank Sloan is the Alexander McMahon Professor of Health Policy and Management and Professor of Economics at Duke University.

Ralph Snyderman, M.D.

Dr. Snyderman is Chancellor for Health Affairs, Dean of the School of Medicine, the James B. Duke Professor of Medicine at Duke University, and Chief Executive Officer of the Duke University Health System.

Louis W. Sullivan, M.D.

Dr. Sullivan returned to Morehouse School of Medicine in 1993, after serving as Secretary of the U.S. Department of Health and Human Services in the Bush Administration. He became the founding Dean and Director of the Medical Education Program at Morehouse College in 1975.

Daniel C. Tosteson, M.D.

Dr. Tosteson has been the Caroline Shields Walker Professor of Physiology, Dean of the Harvard Medical School and President of the Harvard Medical Center since 1977.

Robert Waller, M.D.

Dr. Waller has been President and CEO of the Mayo Foundation for the past 12 years. He is Professor of Ophthalmology and chaired the Department of Ophthalmology at Mayo for 10 years.

Virginia V. Weldon, M.D.

Dr. Weldon is Senior Vice President for Public Policy at Monsanto Company and a past Chair of the Assembly of the Association of American Medical Colleges.

Overview

Ralph Snyderman, M.D.

Our country is undergoing the greatest changes in health care delivery in this century. Therefore, this is an important time to begin a new series of the Duke Private Sector Conferences. The focus of this conference is the academic medical center and how its responsibilities for health care must change to meet rapidly evolving societal needs. This is a critical issue, because academic medical centers play a dominant role in our country's health care system, yet neither the public nor the government fully understands nor appreciates what exactly that role encompasses. Consequently, the viability of these institutions is endangered.

Academic health centers train the vast majority of all types of health care providers. They perform the bulk of basic biomedical research, clinical research, and are responsible for the introduction of new technologies into clinical practice. They care for a disproportionate number of the very ill, indigent, and those with unusual diseases. They are responsible for much of medicine's quality improvement and quality control. On the other hand, academic centers are costly, slow to change, specialty- and high technology-oriented and, as yet, not responsive to many community health care needs.

Increasingly, nonacademic health care providers are competing with academic health centers by delivering good care and excellent service at lower cost. The public, business, and government seem pleased with this trend. As academic medical centers have built educational and research expenses into their clinical charges, they have become too costly and are now heavily dependent on shrinking clinical revenues for academic missions.

Leaders of academic medicine must understand the changing environment and guide the restructuring of their health centers appropriately to enable productive participation in health care reform. On the other hand, the government and the public must understand that academic health centers provide essential national services not available elsewhere. Change is necessary, but academic health centers must educate the public about the need to maintain roles in education and research to improve patient care for the nation's health.

Historical Perspective

William G. Anlyan, M.D.

In 1972, the AMA, the AHA, the AAMC, the Council of Medical Specialty
Societies and the American Board of Medical Specialties established a new fo-
rum for conversation, dialogue, exchange and communication called the Coor-
dinating Council on Medical Education (CCME). I had the privilege of chairing
the group.

The CCME met infrequently in Chicago. From those meetings I got a sense
of how the United Nations Security Council operates, because each of the five
parent organizations had representatives who participated as messengers rather
than decision-makers. It was frustrating because one veto could block a potential advance.

In the final year of my chairmanship, on July 4, 1976, while the nation was
celebrating its 200th anniversary, my frustration led me to write a column about
an imaginary telephone conversation with Dr. Benjamin Rush, whom I presume was in heaven, about government intrusion in medical education and
medical care and the absence of longitudinal memory in the government.

At that time, Alex McMahon, President of the American Hospital Association, and Chairman of the Board of Trustees of Duke University, read this column and wrote to me to ask, "Okay, what are you going to do about it?"

We talked and decided that the time might be ripe (September, 1977) to bring
together on Duke's campus 35 leaders, including those five organizations, private foundations and selected individuals, to establish a dialogue. The 35 people
finally assembled in this building were a heterogeneous group in terms of politics and values.

Over the course of the 2-day dialogue, these people shared meals and conversations and voted to continue the dialogue in about 6 months. We did this for 2
years, every 6 months, and thereafter the group decided to meet annually.

The first published announcement of the group's existence was in *The New
England Journal of Medicine* in 1980. I re-read this report yesterday and was
amazed that the people who were here at that time predicted many of the problems that would be emerging 14 to 15 years later.

Subsequently, we published a monograph on each of the conferences if appropriate, and if not, we published a synopsis. On rare occasions, we decided
that the proceedings did not warrant publication. The books published included: *Health Care for the Poor and the Elderly: Meeting the Challenge; Financing Health Care Competition versus Regulation; Medical Malpractice;*

Physicians & Hospitals: The Great Partnership at the Crossroads; and *How Many Doctors Do We Really Need?*

In 1989, when Ralph Snyderman succeeded me as Chancellor at Duke and Chair of this conference, it was decided to reassess the conference series. I was pleased when Ralph and his staff began to plan for this conference, which takes place in an open atmosphere and requires critical thinking rather than canned speeches.

The Academic Health Center and Health Care Reform, edited by R. Snyderman, M.C. Rogers, and V.Y. Saito. Raven Press, Ltd., New York © 1995.

Session I: The Health Care Environment

Introduction

Ralph Snyderman, M.D., Moderator

During the past few years, managed care has become increasingly dominant throughout the United States. Despite our anticipation that it was coming to North Carolina, the rate of change in our health care market this year has been even more rapid than we foresaw and has been independent of any federal or local legislation. The consumers of medical services are demanding cost-effective health care with an emphasis on cost.

We are entering an era of fundamental change in how health care will be delivered. The core missions of academic medical centers will remain education, research, and health care delivery. However, each of these missions will need to undergo profound revision for several reasons. First, the needs for our services are modifying rapidly. Second, we have new technologies and capacities in all of our core missions that will permit beneficial change. Finally, the sources and amounts of revenues that supported us are changing quickly, and we are facing increasing competition from the nonacademic sector for the delivery of health care services.

Those of us involved in academic medicine, including biomedical research, education and clinical research, believe that the academic medical center must adapt quickly and shape our nation's future health care system. Academic centers need to become more responsive to societal needs and better understand our hybrid structure, which is part academic and part business. We must perform our functions more cost-effectively and size our services to be appropriate to the needs of those we serve. Our centers are threatened, as is the quality of the health care we deliver, and our value is being challenged. To meet this challenge, we must re-evaluate and reconstitute our *modus operandi.*

The Academic Health Center and Health Care Reform, edited by R. Snyderman, M.C. Rogers, and V.Y. Saito. Raven Press, Ltd., New York © 1995.

The Health System as a Mosaic of Cost Centers: The Economic Implications of Health Reform

Uwe E. Reinhardt, Ph.D.

If one had to use a sound byte for health reform, one could probably say that we are attempting to convert the health care delivery system from a mosaic of profit centers in which money comes in every time something is done into a mosaic of cost centers in which every time something is done, money is lost. This stands the economics of health care on its head.

Several forces in our country underscore the need for health care reform. These include:

1. Lack of health insurance for some 40 million Americans at any point in time.
2. Anxiety among the uninsured. (That includes anyone who doesn't have tenure at a fiscally sound university.)
3. Anxiety among private and public payers, not only about the amount of health spending but also over its unpredictability. This item cannot be budgeted for in advance, because actual expenditures will only be evident after a 2-year lag.
4. Anxiety over the quality of health care. (That, of course, astounds those of us who conduct surveys showing that the vast majority of Americans believe we have the best health care system in the world and say, "My last encounter with the medical system was excellent.")

Both the U.S. and Canadian health care systems enjoy high rates of satisfaction; 85% to 87% of survey respondents in both countries rate the quality of care delivered by their health care system as very high. Europeans do not rate their health care systems quite as high.

One of the shortcomings of our health system is that the money flow is splintered in such a way that it is almost impossible to obtain a profile on either an individual doctor—where does his/her money come from and what exactly has he/she done for each patient?—or an individual patient stating the actual health care provided to him/her or to family members. Medicare data files are the only repository of this kind of information, and perhaps one of the reasons physicians fear government control is that it provides transparency.

Peter Welch and his colleagues at the Urban Institute analyzed Medicare data on spending for physician services per the elderly, excluding the effect of age, gender and even the differential prices Medicare still pays, in an attempt to estimate utilization. They did this by approximately 25 SMSAs and reported in *The New England Journal of Medicine* in 1989 that U.S. taxpayers pay doctors $1,800 to take care of the elderly; in Minnesota, only $822; in New York City, $954. One wonders whether these are the correct amounts and what these numbers mean. I do not believe the profession has a good explanation for this, and this is one of the challenges and concerns.

Another concern is the gap over health insurance. It is often said that health insurance is a voluntary and personal choice. When I debated Governor John Sununu, his position was that people choose not to be insured. In my view, this is a matter of choice in the same way that a lot of Americans choose not to drive Mercedes-Benzes.

A prototypical uninsured American family consists of a single mother who is divorced, a secretary, making no more than $20,000 annually, with three children. It is unknown whether her husband supports her. Her situation raises a fundamental question: Why in a rich country, such us ours, should she have to worry about medical bills if one of her children—and they are American kids—gets sick and whether she can afford a doctor?

At a recent conference an economist was asked: Why should the richest nation on earth not be able to afford to give her health insurance? The answer was: Perhaps that is why we are the richest nation on earth.

This powerful doctrine, in fact, drives this debate and will defeat universal coverage. I believe that many Americans who are otherwise of good will fear that whatever is done to provide health insurance for this prototypical woman would wreck our economy, this engine of growth.

Critics of universal coverage point to Europe and say, "Look what's happening to Europe. It is happening because you gave that woman health insurance." Europe-sclerosis couldn't have come at a worse time for health reform and universal coverage. Universal health insurance coverage in the U.S. for that woman does not begin to include the type of coverage that the editorial board of *The Wall Street Journal* enjoys; their employees are covered by a benefit package for vision care, dental care, drugs, and anything else that falls within the area of health care. Yet these are the people who say that Americans are over-insured. The *Wall Street Journal* provides cradle-to-the-grave security for its editorial board, and they write editorials that drive the debate about why this woman shouldn't get health insurance. In my view, these editorials will defeat universal coverage.

A companion theory put forth by many physicians holds that income would have to be redistributed from the top third to the bottom third, roughly $80 billion, to provide this woman with insurance, and that would enmesh government ever deeper into health care. In so doing, this would destroy the marvelous engine of medical progress that American health care represents.

Objections to universal coverage stem from two doctrines, neither of which is economically sound: one is that the welfare state destroys the economy; the second is that government intrusion into health care destroys medical progress. Those two doctrines are supported by at least 60% on Capitol Hill and will defeat universal coverage. We will not have universal coverage in this decade, and it is highly likely that millions of people will remain uninsured in the year 2000.

The amount of money involved depends on the benefit package provided and the subsidies. Roughly, adding $50 billion to national health insurance and another $30 billion to relieve the poor who now do pay for health care would total $80 billion.

Remarkably, that is less than we are already committed to spend for you and me next year. The annual increase in health spending for you and me is larger than it would cost to cover the uninsured.

A report from *Fortune Magazine* showed health spending as a percentage of the gross national product (GNP) from 1970 to 1989. In the 1970s, most nations experienced that slice of the GNP for health care growing just as rapidly and even more so than in the United States. In some ways, and in quite different ways, each country managed to link health spending to the growth of the GNP.

Most economists will state that it does not make sense that health spending should be in lockstep with the GNP. My colleague at Princeton, Bolmar, has written a persuasive paper in which he argues that highly labor-intensive industries, such as education, health care and jurisprudence, which usually don't have the productivity gains seen in manufacturing, generally will see their prices rise relative to the rest of the economy and generally will absorb a larger share of the GNP as the country gets richer, if it is a valid commodity, which health care certainly is.

I believe that a more sensible target for the long run might be GNP plus 1% or plus 1.4%, not GNP plus zero. Europeans and Canadians have shown that you can run for a decade at GNP rates of growth in health care expenditures for a while and survive, but you then defer certain expenditures. In the long run, if you spend GNP plus zero, you would underspend relative to what people would want, if they were fully informed.

If you extrapolate the trend from 1960 to 1985, during which, on average, every year health spending outpaced the rest of the GNP by 3%, into the far future, even at that modest rate from 1985 to now, the differential has been 4%. Thus, the growth of health care costs has been GNP plus 4%.

On the conservative side, with GNP plus 3%, health care alone would take 50% of the GNP by mid-century and 81.5% by the year 3000.

Of the four problems that drove the health care debate in 1992–1993, I believe that lack of universal health coverage is no longer a driving force. Remaining issues include the uninsured/underinsured who want portable insurance that they take from job to job. If that is not provided, there will be continuous clamoring for health care reform. There will be some form of cost control. The issue of quality is already being attacked in a fairly sizable way by the Department of Health and Human Services through the Agency of Health Care Policy Research and by the American Medical Association and the medical centers, who are clearly interested in outcome studies.

To reform the system actually means to redirect the money flow, because we do not do this by edict in this country. Other countries have tried but without success. Ultimately, health reform, even if it is meant to be a reform of the delivery system fiscally, is best achieved by redirecting the money flow.

This is a simplified version of what goes on, but I can simplify this even more by explaining the pie the way an economist might slice it.

At the middle of this process is a collective pot, which could be Medicare, the HCFA, or a company like Prudential. It could be a health alliance, this "farmers' market" for health insurance that the Clintons would like to establish. Whichever it is, the money has to be pumped into that pot and can come only from private households.

In this case, the government can serve as the main pumping station, which is what Canada does, which is what Medicare does; the VA—42% of every American health care dollar goes through this pumping station already. McDermott and Wellstone would like the entire country to be insured through that pipe.

Another option is an individual mandate whereby everyone must buy private insurance, and poor people will receive a tax credit. That would cost between $50 and $80 billion, depending on how high the subsidies are and how generous the benefit package is. One problem with this system is that if the subsidy is taken away as the income of the families rises, low-income families will be quickly saddled with very high marginal income tax rates. Including the loss of health-insurance subsidy, earned income tax credit, and other income taxes they face and maintain the individual mandate that the Republicans favor, it would result in a 70% to 80% tax bracket, which would anger Ronald Reagan because that's anti–supply side.

Therefore, some believe that because there is the problem of a visible transfer from the rich to the poor placing the poor into high marginal tax rates, one could camouflage the whole thing so no one knows. That is called the employer mandate, whereby every employer must offer employees health insurance and pay 80% of the premium while the employee pays only 20%.

Most economists will tell you that in the long run that will get shifted back to the wages of employees. But the employees don't know it, and if they don't know it, we can actually tax these households and make them believe that someone else pays. That adds to the political attraction of the employer mandate.

Another option is a hybrid. An employer with 100 or more employees must offer health insurance; below that threshold, there is an individual mandate, but the government won't finance this, and therefore we will not offer universal insurance coverage this decade.

On the payer side, there are really only two options: (1) fee-for-service, the old-fashioned way; or (2) giving a capitated amount to a private regulator who monitors doctors, the hospitals, and the academic health centers. You can suffer either at the hands of Medicare or at the hands of a private regulator.

The choice from the patient's view is not trivial. Under the old system, a healthy person did not think about doctors and hospitals. When sick, an insured individual had an insurance card and completely free choice of doctor and hospital.

A similar system is used in Germany and Canada, where doctors are bound by a fee schedule. Canadians and Germans have free choice of doctors and hospitals when they get sick.

The approach being propagated in the United States, and into which we will lapse, allows healthy consumers to choose an integrated mini-health care system, a network, an HMO at its best, or some contractual network. When the consumer becomes a patient, he or she will be confined to the doctors and the hospitals in the network.

The Clinton proposal allowed more choice than any other managed care proposal. Under their proposal, the individual would have access to the entire array of HMOs in one's market area. The Clinton proposal would force each plan to have a point-of-service option that would allow a person to buy outside of the plan at a financial penalty, but one could buy out of the plan. Now we have lost this opportunity.

Hewlett-Packard employs a benefits manager who likes two HMOs and, if you want to work for Hewlett-Packard, those are your HMOs—take it or leave it. That's the kind choice Americans will get. It was incorrectly assumed that the Clintons would force the patient to use a government-chosen doctor; that was a lie, and we will pay for this. Choice will be substantially lost relative to the Clinton Plan.

Managed competition, which is bedeviling people on the supply side, is a very simple structure and was described by Insurance Commissioner Garamendi's paper in 1992, which he gave to Clinton and to Ira Magaziner, inspiring them to pursue this route.

Under managed competition, there would be one or perhaps two big health insurance purchasing cooperatives per state. They can be compared to a farmers' market, at which farmers can offer their wares. Here, the "farmers" would be insurance plans. You cannot sell rotten eggs at the Trenton Farmers Market, but, by and large, you can sell whatever you like and grade it any way you want, and you can have unionized drivers or not. They just make a shell available. That's the theory of this health insurance purchasing cooperative, and a model like this is operating in California.

They would offer a booklet listing all the competing health plans in that consumer's area. There might be three HMOs, two Preferred Provider Networks and a fee-for-service plan. The Clintons did say that every alliance must offer a fee-for-service plan unless it's really not feasible. And all plans must bid on a standard package, without which there is no competition because then consumers cannot compare prices.

Here's one package, $100; the other one is $90, but it excludes prenatal care and cholecystectomy. Unless you know that the package is the same, you cannot compare prices. You don't have to make the package as generous as the Clintons did, but there has to be a standard package. Also, these plans would bid on the package at a price per an individual per month. There would be information on each participant in the plan, e.g., patient satisfaction with the doctors and the nurses and clinical outcome data as well. In my view, this is not workable.

If this consumer chooses the fee-for-service plan, all of these plans bid on this package and you will have a weighted average premium bid. The idea of managed competition is that the employer of that individual or family would be obliged to put 80% of the average, not 80% of the premium, into the health alliance and the employee the balance from his or her own pocket into that alliance.

Thus, someone who wants fee-for-service would pay 36% of the premium out-of-pocket; if that person is willing to put up with a low-cost HMO, he or she would contribute only 4%.

It is strongly debated whether the out-of-pocket monies should be deducted from before- or after-tax income. I believe that it should come out of after-tax income, mainly because we need the money to subsidize the poor. If it works, good. If not, nothing was lost. We still have this money. The Clinton Plan stipulated that it should come out of pre-tax income, which was a political decision so they could win approval from the unions and business.

In my view, and probably in the view of most economists, the entire employer provider benefit should be taxed, as the Heritage Foundation and Senator Nichols propose. That would provide $90 billion and he targeted only for the poor.

Now, where does this stand?

Under the Clinton Plan, there would be one large HIPC. Every company, except those with 5,000 employees or more, would have to purchase health insurance through this farmers' market, meaning that 85% of all Americans would be covered.

Some people say they're all in the government plan, and that is either true or false depending on what this HIPC does. If the HIPC is just a farmers' market, then it's not a government-run plan. If, however, the HIPC attempts to regulate, like a farmers' market, you can have only grade A and B eggs, not grade C, and you must use unionized labor for your truckers. If regulation does begin to emerge over the years, then it will become like a department store where you are encouraged to buy merchandise.

People fear HIPCs because no one really knows what this entity is or what it will be like 10 years after legislation. Therefore, I believe that the HIPC cannot possibly survive on Capitol Hill.

Most people would have had to buy through the HIPC, and Medicaid, with its inadequate budgets, would be transferred into it. It would have meant that everyone else would have had to top off the Medicaid patients, which would have raised premiums. We're now getting a bargain from the health sector because we're getting Medicaid patients treated at half-price. If you put them into the HIPC, you've got to pay full price and that has to be paid. Therefore, I do not consider this system of having half-price and jaw-boning optimal.

Finally, large firms could opt out, and the big "rust belt" industries probably would dump their old workforce into the HIPC and pay no more than 7.9% and have the rest of us subsidize General Motors and Ford Motor Company. Companies with young employees would stay out.

Although the Clinton Health Plan died in 1994, pieces of it will survive. The idea of managed competition will survive. Price controls probably won't. Top down budgeting probably won't. The big alliance probably won't.

Universal coverage would have survived if someone had the guts to get $80 billion out of the top third of the income distribution to put it to the bottom. We will have what is called universal access and the pen, the famous pen, will sign universal access, which means we're going to make it affordable and what's affordable will be determined.

We simply declare—like Rockefeller, who declared the Long Island Railroad the best railroad in the world—that health insurance is now affordable and then see whether people will, indeed, buy it.

There will be some insurance reform, but I predict that pre-existing conditions will be excluded. Perhaps there will be a little extra coverage for children and women. Perhaps all people below the poverty line will be insured by Medicaid. But above the poverty line, I forecast very little help in the foreseeable future. I would dearly like to be proven wrong.

If you look at health reform, in 1990, we could have followed the regulated fee-for-service road as in the Canadian model, German model, or Medicare. That would have preserved the independence of the American medical practitioner, even of the surgeon, because he or she could still have a private practice. The medical center would have dealt basically with the government, as they do now with Medicare.

Another option is regulated capitated competition, because it will be regulated regardless. With this route, every year the Congress will add more and more regulation. In fact, originally managed competition was called regulated competition.

U.S. Health Care's unusually rich margin of profits comes from its ability to control doctors and hospitals and other providers. Wall Street cites their loss ratio as 72%, and Wall Street's numbers are the only ones I truly believe. That means for every dollar U.S. Health Care collects, the doctor and hospitals are paid 72 cents, which is high.

Len Schaeffer, a Princeton graduate, and his board members run the Blue Cross Plan in California, non-profit, but they spun off a for-profit subsidiary, 50% of which is owned by Blue Cross, and these people will own substantial stock options that will make them very rich.

Where will they get this money? Not from business, necessarily. They will get it from you. There will be a window of about 10 years during which doctors will be so disoriented and frightened that millions can be made just by scaring them. Eventually, the doctors will wise up and take over the system again. That's what these organizations do. The financial reports on this organization show that the loss ratio is down from 79% to 73%, and the Wall Street quarterly report for the first quarter of 1994 makes it 68%.

In the old world order, which everyone at our previous Private Sector Conference loved, the more a health care deliverer did, the more revenue was made, and profit used to be a fixed cut of that. There was a markup and everyone paid the markup. That's why Tylenol cost $5 apiece, and when a physician administered two Tylenols, he or she made $10 and made the profit thereof.

Now, physicians get the money up front. The idea is to give money up front and then every time a physician does something, he or she loses money. The magnitude of what this will do to the pharmaceutical industry and to the device manufacturers probably has not been fully recognized.

Critics say the pharmaceutical industry makes a lot of money, but they also supported important ventures that we cherish, like *The New England Journal of Medicine, JAMA*, and symposia of various types. Their support will come under siege when companies' profit margins are raided.

I do not understand the economic model of the academic health center. We know that money and real resources go into it, and we value what comes out of it. But we don't quantify what comes out, and therefore it is very difficult for economists to divide the money flow by what is produced to gain some sense of what things cost.

Economists are great cost accountants. We sort out the cost per unit of input or cost per unit of output. But at the academic health center, it comes out in one huge package, and one cannot see where one ends and the other begins.

JAMA says that the faculty:student ratio at a given center is now 1.1 or 1.2 to 1, and many of these people are actually just clinicians. They are the practice plans that bring in the money to support the medical school, but has anyone ever figured out in your centers whether you're actually chasing your own tail?

Support for medical schools has tripled—not academic health centers, just medical schools. Much of that revenue is just practice plan and is needed just to pay the physicians who practice in that plan.

Do we know precisely what the same thing costs now that we did 10 years ago? In other words, the next people you hire probably should not be clinicians, but rather cost accountants and economists who can break this company down into responsibility centers. Then you split that up into service departments and mission departments that bring in revenue by providing services to outsiders. Service departments deliver valuable services, but only to entities within. That is called overhead.

First, you must break your costs into direct costs and into overhead, rather than put this all into one pot, and that is easily done. Then there is overhead allocation. There's direct allocation, step-down reciprocal. We economists don't know how to do this scientifically, or we would call it direct costs. Overhead costs are those costs that you cannot identify with an activity within one of the mission centers. However, many of them can be identified. For example, if you have grounds and maintenance, you can price that out as if it were an outside company and, in fact, you should get bids against your inside grounds and maintenance crew by an outside company. You should always pit your inside service centers against outside service centers so that they perform well. This slicing up of the centers will lead you to a more understandable economic.

Ultimately, education and research are public goods. They will have to be sold to the public sector, because the private sector will not finance them. The private sector will pay for your medical care, but they want this bid.

The other one is, of course, the workforce regulators. There is now a move afoot to regulate the workforce, to regulate how many medical students we allow in residency slots, how many become primary care physicians, and how many become specialists.

I sit on a Physician Payment Review Commission, and the commission endorsed this regulation, but I'm a vocal dissenter. I believe that the market should be allowed to take care of itself. Even with drastic intervention, it would take ages to reach the proper mix of generalists and specialists.

If you see what's happening in the market, you may not actually need all the divisiveness that comes with workforce regulation. In part, we have already tilted the fee schedule substantially in the public sector in favor of primary care.

If the private payers followed the RBRVS, using our conversion factors, primary care physician incomes would increase 43% and specialists' incomes would decrease. Eventually, medical students would notice. Some of us believe that the market could take care of this without setting up an apparatus bound to fail.

There appear to be many demoralized physicians in our country, and I'm astounded how angry even young physicians are because we no longer respect this profession as they still do in Europe and Canada. The old model of medicine was that physicians should decide how to treat a patient and society should respect it. Clinically and economically, whatever you booked, we should pay for it. That, of course, is what gave American medicine its flair for the novel.

Health care is being put into statistical fishbowls, and that is uncomfortable. It is unfortunate that health reform takes place mainly by disorienting what I actually admire as one of the finest professions that there could be. Unfortunately, that is how reform will take place in the 1990s—on the backs of the doctors, making them awfully angry—and we will all pay for that.

The Academic Health Center and Health Care Reform, edited by R. Snyderman, M.C. Rogers, and V.Y. Saito. Raven Press, Ltd., New York © 1995.

Overview: The Evolution of the Academic Health Center in Health Care Reform

Ralph Snyderman, M.D., Moderator

Things are going to be very different for the academic medical center in the years to come. When given a choice, individuals will pay only for what they think is worthwhile. The value of the education and research missions of the academic medical center is difficult for the public to appreciate, and our clinical services are expensive.

If we are to justify government funding for academic medicine, we must make the arguments supporting the value of our core missions understandable and justifiable to the public. We must clarify the value that medical education and research bring to our society. Their present value is difficult to assess.

The public is unaware that the health care field is probably the most dynamic of all enterprises, including the computer industry, microelectronics and space technology. Changes in medical care are driven by discoveries in research and translation into clinical practice. The academic medical center is vital for the continuum of operations needed for quality health care, as well as for future improvements in medicine.

Academic medical centers are responsible for a majority of the nation's basic biomedical research. This largely unfocused research produces discoveries that are identified by other scientists, many of whom are within medical centers, who apply this information to understanding biology and disease. These ideas provide targets for industry to develop new diagnostic modalities or therapeutic interventions. Clinical research, needed to assess the safety and value of new technologies, is done largely within medical centers. In addition, the clinical practice delivered by academic medical centers is often unique in its depth, breadth and complexity and serves the majority of the poor. Outcomes research, the evaluation of what works and what doesn't work, is embedded in the educational and clinical process and keeps progress moving. This continuum from basic research through outcomes research is the heart of the academic medical center (Fig. 1).

Data have been developed that reveal how the core missions at Duke are funded, and they demonstrate the intricacies of cross-subsidization. Though all academic health centers are different, in degrees, we all share similar missions and funding complexities. It will be important for us to identify more accurately

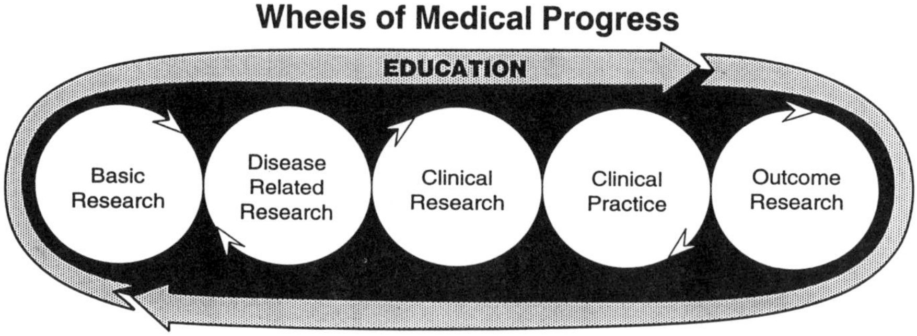

Wheels of Medical Progress

FIG. 1. The continuum of medical progress.

the revenue and expense streams for what we do so that we can understand how we are currently supporting each of our core missions and prepare for change (Fig. 2). Education at Duke University Medical Center incurs more indirect than direct costs. The direct (i.e., faculty salaries) cost of education for our medical students is, at a minimum, $24 million. Revenues (including tuition and alumni support for education) for funding medical education totals $16 million, so there needs to be subsidization of at least $8 million for direct costs alone. Revenues for graduate medical education are also problematic. Our revenues are $32 million, whereas our direct expenses are at least $40 million.

A lot of the revenues for our educational programs are embedded in Duke Hospital charges. This makes them too expensive and noncompetitive in the managed care marketplace. Despite this funding, there is a need for an additional $8 million from clinical practice revenues to subsidize graduate-medical education. For Ph.D. graduate students, the subsidy is at least $2 million more (Fig. 2).

In all, we can account for at least an $18 million direct education deficit, even after factoring in our higher clinical charges and contributions for education from friends of our Medical Center.

Our institution's biomedical research component is the seventh largest recipient of funds from the NIH. Most of our researchers are "well" funded. Nonetheless, an additional subsidization of at least $15 million is needed for our basic research after direct and indirect funding for grants are accounted for (Fig. 3).

Those additional education and research subsidies are largely in the chemical departments and are coming from our clinical practice plan, which last year contributed at least $21 million from a total revenue of just under $200 million. This adds to the cost of our clinical services, yet still doesn't take into account the inefficiency built into our practice as a result of our academic missions. Some of our faculty practice, teach, and conduct research, and one cannot account for the funding of their time very easily.

Figure 4 illustrates how the medical center was doing overall in 1992–1993.

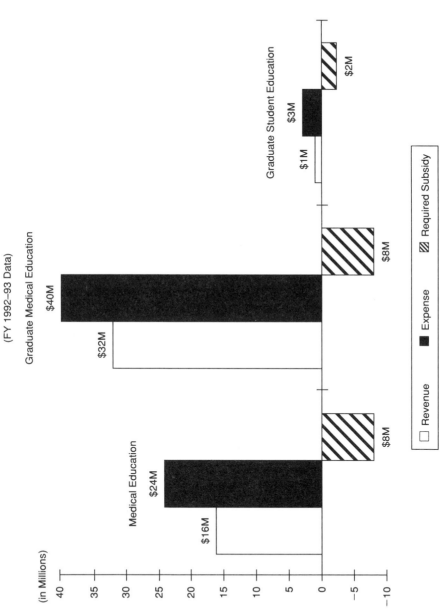

FIG. 2. Clinical income is used to support graduate and undergraduate education.

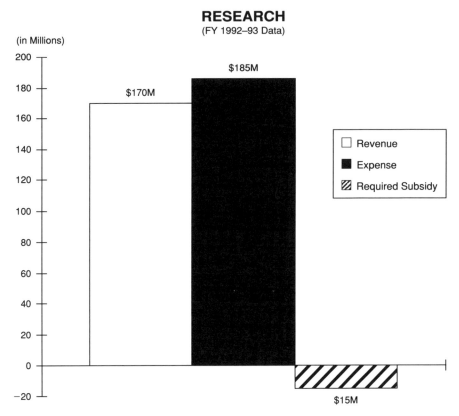

FIG. 3. The research enterprise is not self-sustaining.

The medical school, nursing school, allied health professions, graduate medical education, and basic and clinical research operated at a deficit. This deficit was largely met by dollars from our practice plan, Duke University Hospital, and through support from development. In 1992–1993, we were able to balance our deficit and contribute roughly $50 million to reserves. Considering our revenues of more than $700 million, the contribution to reserves was small, yet this was one of our particularly good years.

A main point for the discussions to follow is: How do we continue to support the academic missions of our medical centers in the face of shrinking clinical revenue margins and increasing competition in our health care markets? It seems clear that our medical centers need to understand better our expenses and revenues and decrease expense where possible. We must understand that we are hybrid organizations—part business, part academic—and act appropriately in each sphere. We must re-evaluate the role of all our core missions in a managed care environment and size them appropriately.

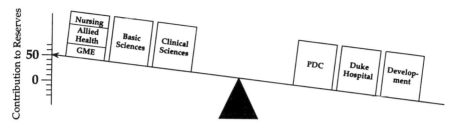

FIG. 4. In 1992–93, clinical income and private giving contributed to the academic subsidy and accounted for $50 million for future program development.

Up until this past year, we could raise the prices for clinical services at Duke University Medical Center to pay for academic deficits and put money into reserves for the future of our Medical Center. Now we are forced to offer heavy discounts for our clinical services. We have no choice but to discount to the level of other providers to retain our patients.

To survive, we believe that we must be prepared to provide excellent care for a large population at a reasonable price while doing outstanding education and research. How do we do this? How do we guarantee that we will have sufficient patients to train our medical students and sufficient revenues to cross-subsidize our other core missions?

The approach that we are taking is multifactorial. First, we must become far more cost-effective in all we do. Needless costs must be expunged from all our activities.

In education, we are reviewing our medical curriculum to enhance our teaching of cost-effective medical practice and to increase ambulatory learning. In research, we are continuing to build our excellence but not our size. We are investing more in the area of human genetics and in neurosciences. We are developing institutional clinical research capabilities and comprehensive clinical and family data bases. In the health care area, we have markedly broadened the primary care capabilities of our practice plan, formed a corporate entity for the purchase of additional primary care practices, and initiated a home infusion company. We are developing capabilities to deal effectively in the managed care environment, and currently we are evaluating the formation of a joint venture to deliver managed care regionally. In brief, we are forming a comprehensive health care delivery network—evolving from a medical center to a health system.

Duke University Medical Center includes a School of Medicine, a School of Graduate Nursing, our hospital and the clinical practice plan (Fig. 5A).

The Duke University Health System now being established will offer comprehensive clinical services throughout our region that will be competitive with

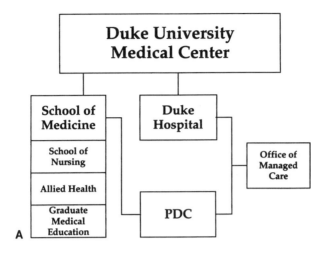

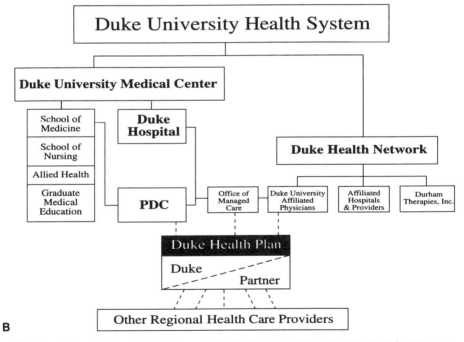

FIG. 5. **A:** Organization of Duke University Medical Center with its educational and faculty practice components. **B:** The Duke University Health System will include a comprehensive health
network and partnership components.

TABLE 1. *Why AHCs are more expensive*

- Cost of medical education
- Cost of intensity of service
- Cost of treating rare diseases
- Cost of introducing new technologies
- Academic responsibilities of clinicians
- Care for uninsured/underinsured
- Inefficient patient care systems
- No prior history of cost-effective strategies

large HMOs and other providers in our area. Our goal is to be able to reinvest a portion of the managed savings from our entity in our core missions. We believe that our institution is capable of behaving in a more business-like fashion and delivering excellent cost-effective health care while retaining our core academic missions and values. We are building a Duke University Health System (Fig. 5B) with a health network comprised of affiliated physicians who provide primary care, affiliated hospitals, home health care, nursing services, and a partnership with a compatible insurer.

Some of the things that will be discussed in this session include the following.

WHY ACADEMIC MEDICAL CENTERS ARE MORE EXPENSIVE

There are a number of things that we can change to become far more efficient (Table 1).

Inefficient patient care systems and no prior history of cost-effective strategies. We need to change that very quickly. Becoming more cost-effective is within the realm of the possible. What we cannot eliminate are the cost of medical education and the added costs of introducing and testing new technologies and our higher intensity service.

The cost of treating rare diseases. There is, for example, not enough clinical volume for pediatric rheumatology in the State of North Carolina to support the clinical programs at Duke, UNC, Bowman Gray, and ECU. However, there is a definite need for care for children with rheumatic diseases, otherwise they won't be treated anywhere. It is the academic medical centers that subsidize the clinical activities.

The cost of introducing new technologies. The costs of medical advances are embedded in our charges. We believe that society ought to be willing to pay for the testing and validation of useful new diagnostics and therapeutics. It is our obligation to make it clear that the challenge of advancing the practice of medicine rests with the academic medical center.

We plan to focus subsequent discussions on where the academic medical center should be going and how we need to behave, both as an academic institution and as an institution that can be competitive with the nonacademic providers that have a different function from ours.

We have asked individuals from government, academic medical centers, and nonacademic health care providers to present their points of view.

The Academic Health Center and Health
Care Reform, edited by R. Snyderman,
M.C. Rogers, and V.Y. Saito.
Raven Press, Ltd., New York © 1995.

All-Payer Funding Stream

Brian Biles, M.D., M.P.H.

My comments will focus on the proposal in the administration plan regarding postgraduate physician training in academic health centers and three themes of the discussion on this particular aspect of the plan.

First, why a proposal for postgraduate physician training in academic health centers? This has not always been viewed as an integral part of health care reform, as proposals for health insurance reform or cost containment for financing sometimes have been. This proposal has been included in the administration plan because officials in the administration wanted to assure the future of the training and quality of care activities of the nation's academic health centers.

The financial status of academic institutions is challenged by the development of competitive health plans. This is a trend, perhaps an accelerating trend, in the current system, as well as one that would clearly be a part of the system envisioned by the administration's plan. The rapid development of competitive plans in the Research Triangle Area in North Carolina indicates, perhaps more strongly than studies or surveys could, that this trend has grown beyond a West Coast or a Minneapolis phenomenon.

If we look at reasons for the proposal, we know that fee-for-service plans over the years traditionally have paid academic health centers 25%–30% more than community hospitals. Competitive health plans seek not to pay any additional costs and particularly these additional costs.

This is important because 80% or 90% of the services that academic health centers provide are bread-and-butter services that can be provided by the larger community hospitals. When Len Schaeffer goes shopping for cheaper services for much of what academic health centers provide, he can find alternative suppliers.

This has led to the proposal to shift funds from the health insurance patient care stream, dollars flowing through Len Schaeffer and all the many insurers, to a single all-payer funding stream. Specifically, the administration proposal would pull funds from Medicare and contributions from all private insurers, and then pay postgraduate physician training and the other activities of teaching hospitals directly on a monthly basis.

The benefits of this proposal are twofold. First, it assures funds for postgraduate training and other expenses often referred to as indirect costs—other training, research, tertiary care—in this case the $9.6 billion in the year 2000. Second, it allows teaching hospitals to price services much more closely in line with community services. Thus, instead of 25% or 30%, the differential would be substantially less. In dealing with plans, the price side need not continue to carry this 25% to 30% differential for both the direct and the indirect costs of training.

The first major issue in the discussion of this proposal is the overall sums. Again, the proposal is $9.6 billion in the year 2000. Many believe that to be inadequate.

In an era of deficit reduction, any expenditure must be balanced with revenues. Revenues mean taxes, and we know how reluctant many members of Congress are to support taxes for any purpose in today's political climate.

The second issue is national goals. The question is: What perceived public need should be met for $10 billion or more of explicit public funds? There has been some consensus for a number of years that a majority of physicians should be trained in primary care. However, there are reasons many people believe the market is unlikely to adjust to this, which are related to issues of cost, quality and availability, particularly in rural areas.

We are now training 70% of new physicians in specialties and subspecialties. The plan provides a gradual shift through the year 2005 to 50%, with some reduction in overall numbers. The shift is managed by private individuals through a national council with a heavy reliance on decisions made in the private sector, either in specialty groups nationwide or by local decision-making groups involving schools and residency programs.

The final point is nettlesome details, involving issues such as what formulas will be used, the duration of transitions, and in what way funds may be allocated. These are all complicated issues and, in an era of change, very important. The committees will probably spend a lot of time addressing them.

There are considerable difficulties in the political debate, and beyond those are difficulties in implementing details year by year. Many people conclude that the better approach to assuring the future of training quality research services is to take the step now to pull this money from its historic base in the clinical-funds flow, ensure that all individuals, whatever their health plan, pay their share, and then attempt to deal as equitably as possible with national decisions in all of these areas.

Committees are discussing these areas, and decisions regarding each of these three issues will emerge over the next few months.

The Academic Health Center and Health
Care Reform, edited by R. Snyderman,
M.C. Rogers, and V.Y. Saito.
Raven Press, Ltd., New York © 1995.

Academic Health Centers Must Undergo Cultural Change

Michael M. E. Johns, M.D.

We have had conversations with many of the managed care entities and large companies. One large for-profit company suggested that it would be a pleasure for them to donate $1 billion to Johns Hopkins University. My interpretation is that they would like to buy us. We need to guard against essentially being purchased over time by for-profit entities that would like to use us as a front and subsequently employ us in ways that may not meet society's needs.

I firmly believe that the academic health centers cannot and will not survive in any useful form unless we have designated public support for the special and vital missions that are part of our health delivery systems. We will not survive if we are forced to compete strictly on a cost-per-patient basis with the HMOs, community hospitals, and providers in the community, unless special funds are made available through an all-payer mechanism to cover the added costs of education, clinical investigation, and the disproportionate share of high-risk patients who seek our services.

We are being asked to transform ourselves and our academic medical centers into health care delivery organizations that can compete on the basis of price and quality (but most likely simply on price, because the quality measurements are still in their infancy), at least for the foreseeable future.

We also will be expected to provide care to populations of patients on a capitated basis, just like everyone else. That requires a radical change in the way we work and the way we deliver health care within our institutions. This entails a substantial cultural change, one that cannot be accomplished simply by a declaration from on high that we will be an integrated multispecialty group practice.

It would be nice, but academic centers have a more complex culture that is well established and not designed to promote unified action. Rather, it is designed to promote diversity, flexibility and individual initiative. This type of organization cannot compete in the new environment.

Our glacial approach will not be satisfactory, and I believe we will have to move much more quickly than ever before. In making these changes, we must remember our research and education missions and the spectacular faculty we have assembled to carry out those missions. We have to make changes without frightening these people away, or destroying their ability to perform their necessary and creative work.

What are we likely to see in our systems? In our faculty and clinical practice, I expect to see a rapid reformation of what are currently very decentralized, turf-oriented entities. They will have to be reformed into an integrated multispecialty group practice in which decision-making is centralized. The departmental interests and individual interests will have to give way to the good of the whole. It will take some skill to make that transition, but many of our institutions, including my own, are well along the way.

The real test of leadership is to evaluate an institution's culture and to determine the right way to engineer the necessary changes. It is our responsibility to articulate a vision compatible with our academic missions that faculty will support.

We are now asking that the leadership of the academic medical center and the departments take a significant amount of responsibility for running a clinical business. We may need different kinds of people to perform those jobs than we have traditionally employed. This does not mean, however, that we want to eliminate the traditional core academic faculty. But we are going to need to identify that core academic faculty, and it will be a smaller group, and clear job descriptions will be needed.

We will need to differentiate that core academic faculty from the core clinical faculty. This new paradigm requires us to have clinicians who are either affiliated with or employees of our integrated delivery system and whose primary responsibility will be high-volume, highly efficient, high-output health care. These clinicians will relate to the core academic mission, but will not be defined by their academic functions.

We will have to put in place all the elements of a delivery system essential for functioning successfully in a capitated market. This means creating a whole new set of corporate entities. The issue is, How do we control them? How do we have oversight of those entities? Do they relate back to the academic mission, and, if so, how?

We've been able to take advantage of the revenue streams from health care delivery to expand and magnify the academic missions. This has had great value to society—creating jobs, new companies, new knowledge. This will continue to be important to the economic future of our country. Now the question is whether the delivery system will continue to support this work.

We have to make new relationships with nontraditional academic health center providers. Perhaps we have been too insular over the past, but I am not sure that we should criticize ourselves with the notion that we haven't done what "society" wanted.

It appears we were doing precisely what society wanted, and we have done it very well. Now society wants something different from us, and we need to be responsive. We need to function differently in the future.

We will need to consider seriously downsizing core academic faculty to match the resources available to support those efforts. At the same time, we need to support the core academic faculty. How do you provide the environment or even the funding for the time for inspiration? How much inspiration time can we actually afford?

That requires a different kind of budgeting. We must have more accountability throughout our institutions. We need to look at program budgeting, and we need to know what people really do. Where do their income streams come from? How do we allocate those streams back, and how do we create accountability?

This will be threatening to our faculties. However, until we can identify what the faculties are actually doing, we will not be able to identify the amount of money that we actually need to fund those activities. This will be a big challenge for us.

At Johns Hopkins, we have been building a new data and information system. We now are loading and tracking data we have never seen before. We can look at the different revenue streams, how much revenue stream is being produced by any individual or any groups of individuals, or combinations or permutations of that. We can also look at how we pay them. Where do the funds come from to support them?

As we explore that, we also get into the issue of effort reports. When I first looked at the system, I hoped to be able to look at Dr. Y and see that 50% of his salary is being supported by clinical dollars and 10% of his income is generated from clinical activity. I should then be able to ask, "Why? Let me see the effort report."

The answer was, "We didn't bother to put in the effort report because it's not really good data." My response was, "We need to put that information in, and it needs to be accurate." We have no choice but to have that information available. It will be a challenge and threatening to faculty, but until we get it, we will not be able to manage ourselves properly.

We need to develop new understandings and agreement with our faculty about what we are hiring them to do. In the past, we have said, "Join the faculty and work hard and you'll eventually be a professor." I do not believe that will work anymore. We will need to state specific expectations, responsibilities, and what we will provide to help them achieve goals we set for them.

We also have to focus on our missions and make sure we are assigning individual responsibilities clearly. We need better systems for evaluating, retaining, and promoting our faculty. We need to re-evaluate tenure. Tenure should probably be eliminated or radically reduced. We ought to begin to look at rolling contracts with a set of expectations and responsibilities. Those could be rolling contracts for different lengths of time, based on different academic ranks.

In addition, we need to look at how we deliver care. We have delivered it by little units and autonomous individuals. We have not delivered it by teams, by interdisciplinary approaches to specialty care, focused on the patient. We have duplicated expertise unnecessarily in clinical arenas. Capitation approaches will force us to change that kind of functioning, which is probably for the better.

We also must devote more attention to the training of generalists and retraining of physicians, but that training is going to have to be radically changed. We hear from managed care companies that today's generalists really are not equipped to work in managed care environments.

One of the issues that has be addressed by medical educators is producing the right number of physicians. Then the focus can shift to the necessary number of specialists and generalists and the issue of distribution.

We must remember that the number of generalists has to have a relationship to the population, not to some percentage of physicians. If there were 50% of a billion doctors, it would simply be too much. From our training in pharmacology, we know that if a 30% solution is the right solution for the body, a 50% solution will poison the system. The idea of overproducing any physician specialty that will result in unemployment doesn't make sense.

We will need to hire more primary care providers within our academic systems and more pure clinicians, and determine how to integrate them and their work as core elements of the institution.

Reassessing the core missions of academic health centers is necessary as well. Can all academic health centers be all things to all people? Or should they differentiate themselves in some way, focusing on different aspects of the mission? I believe that we will have to concentrate some functions and services in fewer centers.

We also will have to investigate creating new revenue streams. Technology transfer and strategic partnering for drug and device development will be increasingly important.

It is important that we remember our accomplishments and how truly exciting the prospects are for the future of medicine. We offer a value system that, in general, is directed at doing well by doing good. That is an important value.

The names of our institutions are generally associated with quality, innovation and integrity. If we look at what we do, we will find that with careful thought we generally can do it right the first time.

We have an advantage in that our physicians are generally employed by the institution and can rapidly reconfigure into multispecialty group practice. We have trained many community physicians, and that could be a nucleus for our physician network.

There is a great need for change and we have many responsibilities, but we also have a great stable of assets upon which to build.

The Academic Health Center and Health Care Reform, edited by R. Snyderman, M.C. Rogers, and V.Y. Saito. Raven Press, Ltd., New York © 1995.

Price Will Determine Our Costs

James E. Mulvihill, D.M.D.

To paraphrase Uwe Reinhardt, we have gone down the regulated, capitated-competition road, and that means managed care and that means capitation. We are now moving away from the fee-for-service, cost-plus reimbursement modalities with which everyone has been so comfortable over the years.

Academic health centers will have to lower their cost structures, if health care is to be purchased in the future on a unit-cost basis, whether it is number of heads (population), DRGs, or other units. In the past, our costs to provide health care determined our price. In the new managed care environment, our price will determine our costs.

In my view, the basis for competition in the future for providing health care will be based on five factors: Price, Price, Price, Service and Quality. Obviously, I believe that price is by far the most important.

Service will be defined by the consumer and the buyer: waiting times, response to a call for an urgent appointment to your faculty practice plan. In the past, the definition of "urgent" for a faculty practice secretary has been, "Well, we can see you in 2 months." That is not acceptable to the patient-consumer.

Quality, which has been a keystone of academic health centers in the past, is important, but I believe it is the least important. In addition, I am not sure that everyone understands quality or how best to measure it.

The measurement of the quality of health services is spawning a whole new industry, not only in academic health centers, but in private corporations as well. Whereas in academic health centers we used to compete primarily on the basis of quality, that will no longer be the basis.

A whole range of relationships will develop through integration, mergers, alliances, networking and affiliations. Insurers may want to relate in some cases to academic health centers, not in a $1 billion takeover or merger fashion, but in a partnership relationship that provides some of the backup processing of information and administration of services—things that many academic health centers are not in a position to provide as they attempt to integrate their systems.

An early good example is the alliance of Prudential with Rush-Presbyterian Hospital in Chicago. The Travelers has explored that possibility, and we have also talked with the administration of other academic health centers, because there are opportunities for partnerships that can benefit the publics we serve.

We will also see more pharmaceutical mergers, similar to that of Medco and

Merck, wedding drug developers and producers with distributors. We have even seen medical schools merge; for example, the Medical College of Pennsylvania has merged with Hahnemann University as part of the Allegheny Health System.

I wonder whether dentistry, which happens to be part of my background, has not done a better job responding to the market than the rest of medicine. A decade ago, there were 61 dental schools, but now there are 55. There used to be 6,500 first-year dentistry students, but now there are only about 4,000. The great success in preventing dental caries through the comparatively inexpensive fluoridation of water has reduced the need for the dentist workforce. This need may increase slightly with our aging population, but it probably will not return to the excessive manpower production levels of the 1960s and 1970s.

Perhaps we should merge some more medical schools. I nearly got thrown off a podium once when I suggested that dental schools in Kentucky merge and noted that 60% of the nation's dental students were educated in only six cities.

On the other hand, because dentistry has never had the revenue flow and income stream from large quantities of NIH, Medicare, and Medicaid money that medical schools have had, it has never had the ability to resist the marketplace quite as much as medical schools may have had.

In the future, we will have to look at partnerships involving the academic health center's dollar and another partner's dollar, whether it is an academic health center with a managed care corporation, a commercial insurer or a data corporation that will help obtain information. Would each of the partners' dollars add up to $3 in community service?

Information is going to be vital, and academic health centers will need sophisticated and highly efficient systems that can produce and process accurate, timely and meaningful clinical, financial, and administrative information at a low cost.

Among other things, this information should enable you and your affiliates to determine the real costs for patient care and teaching, how they are differentiated and distributed across staff, how to price services, how to process the data generated on patients and how to measure the long-term outcomes of care, as well as your variation from standard acceptable practice guidelines and why they exist.

In the future, as a managed care entity or an academic health center, you will have to be one of the top three players in a market to have a successful plan of managed competition with a critical mass of patients and the ability to deliver health services on a price-competitive basis. Can you be, or be in partnership with, one of the top three or four players in your market? If not, you will not last.

Finally, I believe that states will be granted a bigger role in health reform than we might assume. This might cause problems for certain of the private academic health centers left.

If you were governor of a state and had an option under the Clinton plan or any other federally-sponsored plan to do some things to respond to your health and human services needs, you would probably have a single-payer system. Why? Because you could place your insurance commissioner or your commissioner of hospitals and health care in charge of the system. The state agency, functioning as a health purchasing agency, collects the employer and employee health premium dollars. As governor, you tell your agency head to delay the payment for 3 or 4 days, so that the state will receive interest on the float of the premium dollars, which could approach $1 million a day. Over the course of a year, that would be about $360 million the state's governor would have to spend on programs that may not be health-care–related but that may involve other possible health improvements for the public: housing, nutrition, or other social support programs.

Integration as well as the alliances and partnerships within the academic health center are as important as those outside the academic health center. Practice plans need to be examined. There probably will be a shift from the individualistic, capitalistic, departmentalized structures within medical schools to a model that is more like a socialist "kibbutz" or a school-based integrated system.

One of the biggest problems I have observed from within and without our academic health centers is that full-time faculty members often identify more with their national specialty societies than with their department, let alone their medical school or their academic health center. The academic health center must become at least as important to the faculty, if not more important, than the school, department, or the specialty society.

On the question of value, it would be prudent to refine your explanation of your value system to the entities you work with and from which you want support. Your values may not always be understood or agreed upon by members of the academic health community. In addition, the payers may not want to understand them. They already have a lot of other hospitals that offer very good care at lower cost.

They have your fine, educated products as doctors in those affiliated community hospitals providing the care, and they often can work with them more easily than with your full-time faculty. They may still turn to you for the highest level of care, such as the most sophisticated transplant care, something that no one else is doing. That is all they will need you for, and that is how they will interface with you. It will be worth spending the money for a better outcome on a certain kind of transplant, and work with the affiliated hospitals for the other health care they need to purchase, including much of what you define as tertiary care.

Finally, who should provide support? Every entity on the list should help support the unique missions of the academic health center, because academic health centers will continue to be the cornerstone of the advances we make. This applies to managed care entities, commercial insurers and pharmaceutical conglomerates.

Perhaps there is another entity that should also support your academic health center: your faculty. In some cases they may not be doing this to the fullest extent possible. The faculty must understand your uniqueness, your mission and values. The faculty has to be willing to embrace the values and the necessity of supporting the academic health center more than ever in these challenging times.

Until the house gets in order within the academic health center, I am concerned that legitimate efforts to educate the public about your value and about your importance will not be paid attention to by important parties outside the academic health center.

The Academic Health Center and Health Care Reform, edited by R. Snyderman, M.C. Rogers, and V.Y. Saito. Raven Press, Ltd., New York © 1995.

Free Associations

Herbert Pardes, M.D.

I concur with Uwe Reinhardt about the impending "rape" of physicians as one way of correcting the system and to register what I suspect is the concern of many of us. It is not just that the doctors themselves or the profession will be hurt in that process but also the whole process of delivering care will be affected.

Money is not the only determinant for physicians and has not been for decades. I have experienced a collective encouragement for the doctor–patient relationship and the altruism and compassion we all admire. However, I am concerned that money is becoming the dominant issue as we move into a new system.

In my experience, there has never been as high a state of tension in academic health centers as I see now. There are a variety of reasons for this tension.

Scientists in general are in a state of tension and are facing grant approval rates below 20% and in some institutes, even lower. Established scientists are no longer secure. Young people are aware of that insecurity and worry about whether science is the right career choice. This fear is accompanied by a flood of negative science stories that are recurring in the press.

In many ways, all of our scientific institutions are under attack. I believe that medicine, research—almost everything we stand for—is a target for criticism.

People in the academic centers are worried about managed care. They hear the horror stories, perhaps exaggerated, out of the University of Minnesota and of situations in California.

Talk about downsizing and excess supply of various types of physicians, as well as discussions about switches in proportion to primary care, which sound extreme, contribute to the tremendous perception of threat by the collective faculty in academic institutions. Add to that the fact that pharmaceutical companies are somewhat conservative these days in terms of expenditures, as well as the supposed decreased money allocated to biotechnology. Taken together, these factors lead doctors and scientists to believe their autonomy, perhaps even more important than their income, is being threatened. Doctors worry about themselves, their institutions, the way they function.

Examples such as the merger between Hahnemann University and the Medical College of Pennsylvania may be applauded by some and perceived with concern by others. I would argue that the idea of integrations between such organizations is well taken. Within the institutions, the tensions are very formidable.

Hospitals, looking at bottom lines, are confronting academic centers accustomed to working in the academic mode, which means totally different time frames.

Practitioners and full-time faculty are eyeing each other with regard to who should give what to the collective good. As we try to bring doctors together, the people from medicine and surgery and pathology and other specialties are trying to determine how to get one trusted voice. How do we divide money if there's going to be capitated care?

There are other points of tension: hospital workers versus administrators on the one side; layoffs and union people asking why are we paying those high administrative salaries; voluntary teachers saying, "To earn my money, I've got to teach less and, therefore, if you want me to teach, you're going to have to pay me."

Another point of tension involves clinicians versus researchers. When Columbia University recently decided to have a dean's assessment, some of the clinicians suggested that we also try to collect assessments from the researchers, the law school, the journalism school, and every other school on the campus.

The academic health center is basically supported by clinical care and research activity. If you look at the major private schools, somewhere between 66% and 75% of the support comes from those sources. Simultaneously, those of us who work in deans' positions face a steady increase in regulation with absolutely no revenue stream. Other sources of money have various inherent challenges. It is formidable to get anything but restricted gifts from philanthropy.

Regarding indirect costs, the government said we're fat and spending too much, and we could tighten our expenditures. State budgets have been cut. Tuition is decried as being too high. There are few or no opportunities to find capital.

One of the things that gets obscured when we talk about academic health centers or academic medical centers is the medical school part of that center. In discussing clinical care, hospitals leap to mind almost immediately. When we spoke with Mr. Magaziner, we mentioned things like cross-subsidization, the cost of educating M.D.s and Ph.D.s, and the cost of undergraduate medical education and clinical research. I believe these were topics Mr. Magaziner had not heard much about.

New York has not seen the kind of hospital profits that many other cities have seen because it is heavily regulated. A number of New York institutions are scurrying to pick up doctors and hospital affiliations. Affiliations are being made and broken around the clock. For example, Beth Israel, which had been with Sinai, has now affiliated with Einstein. North Shore has broken from Cornell and is joining with NYU.

Obviously, almost any academic health center these days has managed care staffing and an office and is trying to bring together the various constituents within the academic health center, meaning doctors, hospitals, and medical schools.

With the development of outreach clinical facilities, we are converting into more of a system and moving away from what has been a hospital-focused health care enterprise. Active discussion with vendors by most of the institutions is intended to make the system more efficient.

We should consider how we could become more conservative in some of the recruitment packages that bring faculty from one institution to the other. We are working on ways of maximizing other streams of income.

I also believe that cross-institutional collaboration with economies and regionalization is one of the other orders of the day. Obviously, we are in the business of substantial curriculum change, trying to encourage greater attention and modeling for primary care and encourage general practice.

In closing, I consider it rather remarkable that two of the most productive and successful institutions in this country—my bias is obvious—are the NIH and the academic health center. They are not perfect, and they have all kinds of problems. We should consider why these two institutions are in the kind of trouble they are in, given the general view that they are valued institutions in this society.

The Academic Health Center and Health Care Reform, edited by R. Snyderman, M.C. Rogers, and V.Y. Saito. Raven Press, Ltd., New York © 1995.

Responses

Frank A. Sloan, Ph.D.: On two occasions in the past, I've undertaken an analysis of why cost per case varies across hospitals. When this is done, depending on what factors are adjusted for, the major teaching hospital costs about 25% to 30% more than community hospitals.

In analyzing this differential, an attempt is usually made to include some case-mix variables, but there is something that we aren't really catching, which I call unmeasured severity. Then there is teaching activity and unsponsored research.

Regarding quality, some evidence indicates that the quality of major teaching hospitals is higher, not nearly as much published work as there ought to be.

Severity is a crucial issue. Some of my colleagues say that they do not believe that we can develop a severity measure for the risk before the case is handled and the cost of that additional risk. Obviously, that would be critical for an academic health center that attempts to treat more severe cases, as well as cases that aren't so severe.

Then there is the issue of teaching activity, and there will be plenty of public debate over whether it can be done less expensively.

In the future, it appears that individual centers will need to develop measures of quality and demonstrate that they can deliver a quality product. It will no longer be sufficient to say simply that we do a better job. It might be hard to demonstrate quality for individual centers because often large samples are required, but certainly it is manageable for groups of centers.

Measures of severity of illness need to be refined. This work has been done largely by people at HCFA and by a few researchers. Fine-tuning these measures offers an excellent opportunity for clinicians, economists and others to work together. Payment can then be based on these measures or for other reasons as well.

Other challenges we face are the high-cost cases that the HMOs will not want. One of the big problems with capitation is the severely ill person with many long-term problems. This is not the kind of patient that many HMOs will want to enroll. If we could determine a more efficient way to care for this kind of patient, it could be marketed to HMOs and others.

In my view, there is an argument for public subsidy of teaching, as there is for unmeasured severity and high severity. There is no way for the centers to survive without a subsidy.

Unsponsored research is the hardest to defend probably of all the pieces, but fortunately is not a big piece.

32

Louis W. Sullivan, M.D.: There is no question that academic health centers play a very important role in generating the values in our health care system. We now face a change in our environment that demands dramatic changes in the academic health center.

Most of our discussion has been about cost of care in academic health centers, concerning how we organize, deliver and pay for health care. I believe that the academic health centers of the future also will have to work to change the health behavior of our citizens.

During my time as Secretary, I visited other countries that had much lower health care costs, and the health status of their citizens was as good as or better than that of Americans, particularly in terms of infant mortality and life expectancy. Japan is a remarkable example, because it spends about half per capita of what we spend for health care, yet has a lower infant mortality rate and a higher life expectancy than we do. Also, their society experiences much less violence: There are more murders in Washington, D.C., every year than there are in all of Japan.

Our Public Health Service has estimated that if we could change the health behavior around the top ten causes of death in our society, we could reduce premature deaths, i.e., before the age of 65, by a minimum of 40% and possibly as much as 70%. Equally striking is the estimate that we could reduce acute disabilities in our society by one-third and chronic disabilities by two-thirds.

What all of this means is that we have to emphasize those behaviors that keep people healthy, out of hospitals, out of doctors' offices. The academic health centers will have to take a leadership role in this effort. If we focus only on what needs to be done once illness or injury occurs, then academic health centers rapidly will become obsolete.

The shift to greater emphasis on ambulatory care, on community clinics, and toward primary care physicians is part of this effort. An important role for academic health centers is to help us find ways to educate our citizens about improved health behavior.

We need to find ways to improve our ability to reach low-income and minority populations. Two studies in *The New England Journal of Medicine* in May 1993 pointed out that the gap in health status between the poor and the affluent in the United States has widened over the past 25 years, despite all the funds we have spent on health care.

These articles also pointed out that in England, a similar widening of the gap in health status between affluent and poor had occurred. To me, that means that universal access to health care does not guarantee improved health status. We have to find more effective approaches to address that gap.

In addition to the sophisticated high technology complicated care that academic health centers provide, they will have to develop approaches to working with community physicians, lay people, and the business community to improve the health behavior of our citizens. If this isn't done, it won't matter what kind of reforms we enact—we still will be faced with escalating costs far beyond what we can afford.

One of the perverse outcomes of first-dollar coverage, in addition to other actions, has been to insulate individuals from the cost consequences of their decisions. Consumers themselves have to become more conscious of the financial consequences of their decisions as another measure for cost containment.

Robert Waller, M.D.: Someone mentioned earlier: Price–Price–Price. For our future, we see Expenses–Expenses–Expenses. But most importantly, Value–Value–Value, which is a function of quality, appropriateness, and price.

We have been following the growth of national health care spending per capita, which Uwe Reinhardt estimates to be around 5.2% inflation adjusted between 1988 and 1993. In our particular health care system, our rate of growth and expense per patient has been about 1.2% during that period.

At the Ways & Means Committee testimony not too long ago, we were asked to comment on the difference in these two growth rates. The tongue-in-cheek answer was that we were predominantly fee-for-service; we were composed mainly of specialists; we took care of increasingly sick patients; and we invested heavily in research and education.

In point of fact, fee-for-service payments in many systems are disbursed to employees on a salaried system. We have no bonus or incentive plans in our compensation programs.

Our specialists, as is true in many places in this country, provide general care in addition to their specialty practices. Efforts are made to accomplish much of diagnostic and treatment plans in outpatient settings. Finally, the major goal is to practice medicine within a broadening spectrum of inquiry, including basic research, bench-related clinical research, human protocols, technology assessment, continuous improvement, outcomes research, and practice guidelines. Hopefully, these activities add to the value of services.

It is encouraging that the integration of Mayo Clinic, St. Mary's Hospital, and Rochester Methodist Hospital into one organization has allowed us to reduce overhead expenses significantly in several areas. This is perhaps the leading factor in reducing our costs of care per patient registration in recent years.

We closed one emergency room and one catheterization lab. Most of our support services have been consolidated. During the past 9 years, we reduced the equivalent of about 750 beds in our Rochester hospitals.

We're about the business of building an academic health system, as David Blumenthal described in *The New England Journal of Medicine*. For us this means the medical center on the one hand, a host of new partners on the other, and electronic data interchange to link us all together.

Several years ago, our trustees concluded, rightly or wrongly, that there would be few dollars for research and education from the practice of medicine in the decade ahead.

We have taken the position that long term, the practice must sustain itself. We define "practice" to include support for residency and allied health training, working capital and inflation-adjusted depreciation. We hope that an enhanced fund-raising effort, as well as seeking revenue through a variety of activities we call "diversifications," will in the future support the medical school, the graduate school, continuing medical education and Mayo-funded research.

We believe that it will be exceedingly difficult for us and other academic health centers to predict future revenue.

Virginia V. Weldon, M.D.: What can academic medical centers learn from American business? What are the factors in the academic medical center that make it so difficult for them to fit into an economic model that they're being pushed toward?

The factors as I see them are that academic medical centers are part of an overall complex system of health care delivery, and they are linked to each other in ways that most businesses are not: through the specialty societies and specialty boards. They recruit each other's faculty with an openness and at a slow pace that is unknown in industry.

Academic centers have been constrained from responding quickly to change by their traditions and by these linkages that keep them from being truly free-standing from each other. Also, academic centers are part of an economic model in which the customer doesn't pay the bill.

All of those factors make it difficult for academic medical centers to think about change in the same way that an American company, or a multinational or global company considers change.

The merger mania and the takeover artists of the 1980s are given credit for setting the stage for the change that most American companies are experiencing right now. America has been at the forefront of recognizing that many companies had lots of opportunity to cut costs and do business differently.

During the past 8 years, Monsanto has gone through a number of change activities that could be applicable in some ways to academic medical centers. The first area is cost reduction. We have looked closely at how we do business, including details such as our order entry forms, how we deliver products to customers, and how responsive we have to be.

We have reviewed the portfolio of the businesses we own and our company has down-sized from 60 businesses to 12 businesses today; we are in the process of acquiring three new businesses. We had 60,000 employees 10 years ago, and now we have 33,000 employees.

We have re-engineered many of our businesses from top to bottom. For example, our chemical company does business now in a completely different way than it did 10 years ago. The kind of people we employ are different. They must be flexible and able to adapt to change.

The head of General Electric, Jack Welch, has told employees that he will not guarantee lifetime employment, but he will guarantee that they will be employable for their lifetime. That is a very different message from what most major corporations gave their employees just 10 years ago.

We cannot apply the lessons learned in industry blindly to academic medical centers, or we will lose some of the values and traditions that are most important and that have made academic medical centers great.

The Clinton Health Plan is a wake-up call for our academic medical centers, just as the corporate raiders of the 1980s were a wake-up call for American companies. We cannot continue to do business in academic medical centers the way we have done in the past.

The Academic Health Center and Health
Care Reform, edited by R. Snyderman,
M.C. Rogers, and V.Y. Saito.
Raven Press, Ltd., New York © 1995.

General Discussion

Dr. Anlyan: I would like to ask Uwe Reinhardt about the Federal Employee Plan and why that isn't being considered to cover the uninsured.

Professor Reinhardt: That proposal led many of us to think that the Clintons may have taken on too much. It may have seemed reasonable a year ago, although many of us have doubts.

I published a plan that proposed leaving the private sector alone; just see where it leads. The uninsured would pay an income tax to a federal fail-safe pot that would be supplemented with a tobacco tax, phasing in taxes on employer-provided benefits for people earning more than $35,000. This plan would have amassed $50 to $60 billion. Then several things would have been possible.

It could have been called Medicare. Or the Federal Employee Benefit Program could have been made available for the purchase of health insurance through it, or it could have been capitated it to the state.

Had the Clintons done that in March of 1993, we might have had universal coverage. In the meantime, they had this huge task force, frightened and angered many people, and we are in the current situation.

That idea is not bad, which is why Senator Nichols' plan using that kind of mechanism is worth considering, even though it hasn't received much attention from the press.

Dr. Joseph B. Martin: Dr. Waller, please expand on your comments that there would be no dollars, as I heard it, from clinical practice for research and education.

Dr. Waller: We do not expect many dollars from the practice of medicine to sustain our programs in education and research. Medicare patients represent approximately 40% of our practice. The Medicare program has clearly benefitted our older citizens, but Medicare price controls have had a significant impact on our revenues. The impact on our system in 1994 is projected to be a negative $83 million.

We see private payers seeking Medicare payment rates (or less). We also see enormous pressure on our revenue streams from every angle, and we must find nonclinical revenue sources to sustain our programs in research and education.

Dr. Arnold Relman: I concur wholeheartedly. I am interested in your statement that your trustees made this decision 10 years ago. At that time, I gave a speech at the Association of American Physicians on the financing of clinical medical education, stating that we had been through a period in which we tried to bootleg the costs of medical education from research overhead. That clearly wasn't working. Now we are trying to find out whether we could bootleg it through clinical practice plans. That clearly won't work either.

There is no way we can pay for the cost of education if our students can't pay for it, except through earmarked funds.

Dr. Thomas W. Langfitt: I've been thinking about how academic health centers are going to become better organized, more efficient, and more productive. People from academic health centers around the country are thinking about this, but I have a strong sense that many of them are uncertain about what to do. At this point, health centers are going to need a lot of help, and the question is where to turn for that help.

The leadership of the academic health centers could turn to both the service side and the industrial side of the corporate sector. Many corporations were in far poorer shape than anybody thought, and they have undergone fundamental reform in the past several years and emerged much stronger.

Before restructuring, for a long time many corporations faced the same problems that we in academia face. It was difficult to get organized and to develop a mission that everyone could understand. There was a tremendous amount of autonomy within the units of the corporation, just as there is within academic institutions. Of course there were cost centers, but no one paid much attention to them.

That has changed in a fundamental way over the past decade, particularly in the past 5 years, and was driven by the same pressures that drive the academic health centers today—namely, a constraint on revenues.

Dr. Mark Rogers: The question we face does not seem to be whether there will be all or none in terms of support for the research and teaching missions coming from clinical care. The real question appears to be whether there will be sufficient funds for us to be able to continue the expectations and the culture of the academic medical centers.

We have two things to think about. One is what we can do in competition with those for-profit organizations. We must come to grips realistically with how much money we put into this. Also, we must understand the enormity of the task of replacing our clinical support for research and education.

Ralph Snyderman mentioned earlier that we were putting $50 million into reserves. Everyone here understands that if that is true, it is a gross underestimation of the transfer of funds that occurs in an institution like this.

It does not address how we pay clinically competitive salaries to physicians who spend 85% of their time in research. It does not address putting together competitive packages to attract people. It also does not address a large amount of clinical funds that end up indirectly supporting basic sciences, causing people to say the issue is about downsizing.

Using different cost accounting methodologies, I estimate that we reinvest between $100 and $150 million of our expenses in this institution, and similar percentages in your own institutions that are transfers from clinical work to support the infrastructure of buildings and people.

I contend that the kind of business we are entering will not allow us to take $150 million out of $750 million of revenue and to call that "margin" and pay clinicians.

Dr. Johns: Dr. Waller, you mentioned development and investment of your cost and diversification of other areas may be your sources for funding those missions, but there may not be enough money to fund them at the same level. Have you thought into the future about that?

Dr. Waller: Yes, we have. Mayo Medical Ventures has been in existence for 8 years now; its sole purpose is to generate alternative sources of capital to help support our academic missions. Mayo Medical Ventures has four divisions: technology transfer, medical products, health information for the public, and a new ventures division.

We will need to accelerate our efforts to keep up with our growing needs. We are also looking at enhanced fund raising efforts and are encouraged that there may be growing interest in supporting endowment funds as well as capital for construction. I would like to know whether The Duke Endowment and others are finding this to be true as well.

Hopefully, society will recognize that investment in research and education is to everyone's benefit and will find a way to fund academic missions through legislation. We cannot be certain about this latter possibility, so we believe we must try to put other plans in place.

Dr. Weldon: I think Thomas Langfitt had a good point. One of the things you would learn from American corporations and their consultants is the pace at which the change has to take place. We can't wait 10 years more for that change to take place.

We also need to think about whether our students are going to be able to afford their education. A faculty:student ratio of 1.5:1 strikes me as a very expensive educational system. We have to examine the true costs of education and determine whether we can reduce them.

Dr. Pardes: Dr. Langfitt, please elaborate about corporations and academic health centers being comparable. One of the most formidable problems for leaders in academic health enterprises or universities is a tradition of consultation–involvement–democratic decision making. Unless Deans were to become dictators with absolute power, I am interested in the ways in which we must move, as corporate America may have moved.

Dr. Langfitt: We all recognize that the corporate culture and the academic health center culture traditionally have been fundamentally different, and they have different missions. But we're no longer talking about academic institutions in the true sense of the word. As academia moves in the corporate direction, there will be a cultural change.

It is a tremendous challenge to the leadership to try to move the troops in that direction. The only good news about all this is that perhaps, for the first time, we really have their attention.

Chairman Snyderman: That's a key point. Here at Duke University, it has taken us several years to understand what we need to do to act as a corporate entity, and we are beginning to have a vision of that. We have just begun to develop the governance mechanisms to allow our institution to act more effectively. The greater challenge for us is to get sufficient buy-in through the University so that we can actually do what we need to in a timely, coordinated manner.

Professor Reinhardt: The point was raised that the centers may not have the capital to accomplish some of their goals. People say we need access to the capital market, but we really don't want to soil our hands, so why don't we have a for-profit subsidiary and let that have access to the capital market.

This is a slippery slope to go down. You will have to compensate those people the way their peers are paid, $1 million or $2 million with stock options, and that will demoralize the faculty.

Dr. Relman: Are you really recommending to academic health centers that they go into public capital markets?

Professor Reinhardt: No. I predict that academic centers could certainly explain to society or the Congress that there isn't enough public support for the valuable things that they do. Their accomplishments have market value.

Dr. Relman: The Newt Gingriches and the Phil Gramms in the Congress would say, "Fine, that's exactly what you ought to do!" Don't we want to have some values and ideas of our own as to what really would be in the best interests of American society?

Professor Reinhardt: The temptation to do that is more than just the fantasy. I think I could really see that.

Dr. Mulvihill: If one of your missions is research, you have researchers on your own faculties in many health centers in this country who have already gone even further in their interactions with the private sector and corporations than we are discussing here.

Are you looking for a model in which patient care affiliations with managed care entities support the academic health center and still preserve your values? This is similar to what some of your faculty have done individually as they have interacted with corporations and biotechnology venture firms.

For example, I could see a Duke University Health System lacking some capital, initially turning to partners in the private sector who can generate clinical and other outcomes information. Perhaps the academic health center would turn to managed care organizations or commercial insurers or to other for-profit health care companies for a partnership that would set up a regionalized health network in the area.

It would attract dollars, perhaps enabling you to meet your need for more primary care practitioners and to support education. What's wrong with a managed care company wanting to invest in helping to support the primary care residency?

Dr. Johns: Insufficient capital is a major problem for us. We cannot generate huge amounts of capital through the hospitals providing $50 million profits or by any of the other mechanisms that we have used in the past.

This issue of going public needs further discussion, because it is one source of capital required for us to be competitive. We have a number of other entities already doing this and doing it very well.

U.S. Health Care and some of the other publicly traded companies are successful and in many ways more successful than Prudential, the Travelers, or any company. They are focused on one product line that just happens to be hot. Through the public marketplace, they can generate the capital to get it done. I believe that U.S. Health Care has $1 billion capital, as does United.

What we have is a pittance next to that. Setting up a primary care physician network will cost $200,000 to $300,000 a practice; you may need 500 primary care physicians in your network, and you want them to work in a different way now. You don't want them to be faculty or teachers. You must be able to buy those practices and set them up properly, with appropriate information systems in place.

I estimate the need for $50 to $100 million merely to establish a primary care physician network, and possibly another $50 to $75 million to build the information system and financing system to track the data.

I agree that you could seek partnerships, but it may not be easy to find partners. There's a primary care physician business called Health Spring, which is a Warburg/Pincus/Styron venture group. There is venture capital money creating physician groups in various cities. In Philadelphia, a lot of money has been raised through venture capital.

We have been considering this option for Johns Hopkins, because we know that the capital is critical. We are being forced to create a system to deliver health care that requires huge amounts of capital that we just don't have.

Dr. Relman: Even more fundamental than the question of how to pay for medical education is confronting how we want to regard our health care system. Do we want to fold it into the American economy and turn it over to business and venture capital and operate it the way that most of our economy is operated, or do we want to retain it as something quite different?

We haven't come to grips with that yet as a society. If you believe that health care is just another part of the American economy, then the question is how to be efficient and reduce costs and generate the capital needed. If we follow that route, we will end up in 10 or 20 years with a sorry excuse for a social system of the sort that health care ought to be.

Now is the time for us to determine how to move in the other direction. It can be done, because the money is there. We are spending the money now, but the money is disbursed through inappropriate channels, and is controlled by inappropriate management. We are watching the hundreds of billions of dollars on American health care go through corporate America with a 29% or 30% rip-off of the top.

There is plenty of money to provide the necessary capital and for research and education if we used it in a different way. That probably is politically impossible now, but I believe that we are closer to the cutting edge, to the business part of this machine than anyone else. We ought to try to convince the public and the government that there is a better way to use all that money.

Dr. Pardes: When economic or business forces start to influence prominently the character of the institutions in this enterprise, then one has to raise questions such as: Do things like academic freedom reconcile comfortably with that? Should we rewrite the Hippocratic Oath? Are we going to change dramatically the character of individuals who want to go into this enterprise?

Many of us within academic medicine may understand the nature of this enterprise, but I believe if we were to decide that academic medicine should retain some special character, we would have a formidable challenge explaining this in understandable and convincing ways to the average American citizen.

Chairman Snyderman: A critical question is whether the academic health center could be out in front and use the appropriate margin to sustain the core missions—is this the kind of business we are contemplating?

Dr. Daniel C. Tosteson: We are looking at a redrawing of the interface between the medical industries on the one side and the medical profession on the other (not limited to academic medicine). It is a fundamental examination of the relationship of the physicians and other medical professionals to their patients on the one side, and the emergence of the complicated corporate structures required to deliver modern medicine to patients on the other side.

Dr. Roscoe R. Robinson: Access to capital is a problem. My own institution is exploring the feasibility of some of the approaches discussed today, and I believe that there is a middle road. For example, we have at least one for-profit company that is a wholly owned subsidiary of my university. We haven't even begun to think about taking it public, but such an approach in the future is not without possible merit. The cost of efforts to restructure our delivery systems via networking, partnering, alliance building, and right-sizing will be very high, so access to adequate capital is of paramount importance if we are to preserve those high standards and other missions that we value so highly.

It is said that the major drivers of increased cost can be attributed to such things as "increased morbidity due to good medicine" and "an ever-expanding definition of health." We are now adding the adverse consequences of violence to that definition.

I would like to know why the free marketplace doesn't seem to work well in pricing high technology in health. Competition-induced price reduction in the sale of common household appliances is often associated with the delivery of improved products, but slight improvements in life-saving, high-tech equipment are often associated with higher pricing. I have never completely understood that phenomenon.

Tremendous marketplace opportunities have been produced by our attempts to control cost via the behavioral regulation of medical practice. Short of global budgeting, I don't know of a single western country that has attempted to control costs by the behavioral regulation of medical practice. We are measuring outcomes and quality; we are doing pre-certification and utilization review, and we are developing and monitoring best-practice guidelines—all this is enormously expensive.

Do I see an opportunity here for third parties? Of course, if I am an opportunistic entrepreneur I will tell you that I can help to make it operate better, and that you will have much more time to see patients and issue more charges. The patients will come and, simultaneously, as you practice, I will handle all your claims processing and other administrative tasks. But, between your increased billings and my addition of another mouth into the system that will have to be fed, the aggregated cost of health care goes up.

I am not persuaded that the advent of a plethora of market-niche administrative services, with their supposed increases in task efficiency, has driven total cost down as opposed to driving it up.

It is true that we must reduce both our unit and total costs. Our own hospital has been working hard at this for the past 3 years. Our billable charges today are 6% below their level in fiscal 1991 and our costs per discharge in the first 9 months of this year are up 0.6% over last year. We are beginning to make real headway in the reduction of hospital billings and cost.

In hard dollars, we have taken almost $30 million out of the expense side of Vanderbilt Hospital in the last 3 years. We've put in self-developed computer software programs for the management of some 300 diagnoses on several inpatient units. They are our variant of best-practice guidelines, developed through collaborative efforts between nurses and physicians.

Several such approaches are already being implemented in the private sector without governmental intrusion. However, if I were to give the current administration any credit, I would have to say that it has attracted my full attention in a way that has not been equaled thus far.

Mr. McMahon: There is another side and, before you take that easy road, you ought to explore it very carefully. If you take out the health system or the educational system or any system from the regular part of the economy, then you have to put it in the hands of the government. The leaders of the government are going to come out of that same entrepreneurial side that you want to avoid. I do not believe they will deal with you gently. They will be worse than the entrepreneurs themselves.

Dr. Relman: I side with those who say we should not socialize our health care system, and we should not have government own or control it. The question is: Is it possible to have tax-supported health care that is delivered and organized and managed locally? It would be in the hands of communities and the professional health care givers, the hospitals and the doctors and the nurses. Or is that a mirage?

Mr. McMahon: It is a mirage because there is no way to get the U.S. Congress to raise money and to turn it over to someone else to spend. If they raise the money, they will dictate how it is to be spent, and therein lies deeper tragedy than what we would have if we were to go another route.

Dr. Mitchell T. Rabkin: Without diminishing the importance of these points, I believe that one has been overlooked. Brian Biles pointed out that there was $9.6 billion, representing recognition by the government that teaching costs were valid to support. How does that $9.6 billion come about? That $9.6 billion is projected to the year 2000, as I understand it, and inflated to the year 2000.

It comes out of two things. One is the IME, the so-called Indirect costs of Medical Education, calculated at $5.3 billion in 1991, and that alone projects to about $9.2 billion in the year 2000. The other is DME, Direct costs of Medical Education, where the average cost per resident is multiplied by the number of residents. That was about $3.6 billion and was projected to the year 2000 to about $4.8 billion. The total of these two projections is $13.8 billion, the amount that today's payments project to the year 2000.

So you might say, there's $9.6 billion available, and that is, in fact, 70% of what you are getting now. There is enough fat in the system so you ought to trim it. And everyone will agree to tighten our belts.

However, this starting figure of IME—Indirect Medical Education—of $5.3 billion does not actually relate to what we are getting today. The actual IME today is calculated at 7.7% rate in relation to the number of residents. But when HCFA came up with a projection on that basis, someone said that amount should actually be 3.3%. Instead of a figure projected to $5.3 billion, the actual projection on the basis of today's IME payments is something like $12.4 billion. Somehow this step of going from $12.4 to $5.3 billion seems taken for granted.

Instead of saying, "Look, we expect you to clean up your act and make do with 70% of what you're getting today," the IME projection turns out to be something like 38% of what we're getting today.

It is critical to review some of the basic assumptions that underlie good motivation on the part of the government to recognize teaching costs and to make sure that they understand that you simply cannot say, "You really ought to tighten up your act. We're going to give you 38% of your salary next year, but we're going to call it 70%."

The Academic Health Center and Health Care Reform, edited by R. Snyderman, M.C. Rogers, and V.Y. Saito. Raven Press, Ltd., New York © 1995.

Session II: Are the Missions of the AHC Relevant to Society?

Overview

Arnold S. Relman, M.D., Moderator

The questions that we are currently dealing with are long overdue: When and how will the missions change? What does the academic health center do that is unique? How can it become a model for cost-effective care of continually improving quality? What services should it provide? What should it not do? If we had acted intelligently, we would have asked ourselves these questions years ago when it became apparent that we were spending at a rate that needed to be curtailed. The revolution in health care has made it urgent that we address these questions now.

The revolution and the organization of health care is the conversion from a fee-for-service indemnification kind of payment to capitated prepayment and organized systems—managed care. It appears that this process of change is taking place inevitably and will not be affected significantly by legislation coming out of the Congress this year.

The Academic Health Center and Health Care Reform, edited by R. Snyderman, M.C. Rogers, and V.Y. Saito. Raven Press, Ltd., New York © 1995.

Looking to the Corporate Sector

Thomas W. Langfitt, M.D.

Two powerful sets of forces, largely independent of each other, are afoot within the health care system. One is in the private sector, which is probably going to be the most important force in terms of the academic health center. The second is the actions of federal and state governments.

All academic health centers in the country will face these forces within the private sector, which focus on competition for patient revenues based on price and perceived quality. To respond, almost all academic health centers need to develop a vertically integrated patient care system or, to use another term, an accountable health plan.

The system needs to incorporate a strong primary care base that includes physicians and other health care providers. It also should include an assortment of community hospitals, providing specialty care such as rehabilitation and long-term care. The one or more tertiary care hospitals within the system must not be allowed to dominate it. The academic health center should then link up with an insurer so that insured patients who provide the revenues are brought within the integrated system.

This kind of accountable health plan is not responsible for all patient services provided by the academic health center, but it becomes the core. The institution continues to contract with other insurers and to operate fee-for-service practices but has a substantial patient base to rely upon through its contract with the large insurer. Some of the large insurers have fairly deep pockets, and they might be able to provide capital needed by the academic health centers.

A set of values defines the academic health center that has nothing to do with business. These values frame the responsibilities and quality of patient care, the education and training of health professionals, and the research mission of the institution. They need to be protected from economic forces. Because of the enormous power of commercial forces, the academic health center will not have the opportunity to preserve those values, functions, and missions unless it is able to survive, and indeed thrive, in this new environment.

The Academic Health Center and Health
Care Reform, edited by R. Snyderman,
M.C. Rogers, and V.Y. Saito.
Raven Press, Ltd., New York © 1995.

Competition in a Changing World

Steven A. Schroeder, M.D.

As I hear the anguished cries of those entrusted with trying to guide academic medical institutions in these very difficult times, I sense the dilemma, because everything has been fine until now for many of the faculty. They have been buffered from many of these changes. Academic leaders are responsible for letting the faculty know that things are changing, but it is difficult to communicate that message. If the messenger is too visible, the temptation is to criticize the messenger, not the message. On the other hand, if the messenger is too far behind, he has lost the game.

The answer to the question, "Are the missions of the academic health center relevant?" is, "Of course." However, there is tremendous heterogeneity among the 126 plus academic health science centers in the United States. This is not just a difference between Washington Heights and Durham, or whether or not an institution has a Dean's tax. It is difficult to have a uniform posture regarding the requirements of academic medicine, because, as someone said, "If you have seen one academic medical center, you have seen one academic medical center."

The first of the three major missions of the academic health center is research. The public is willing to spend tax dollars on research, because it is desirable to find a cure for Alzheimer's disease, AIDS, or cancer. In fact, research is one of the few areas of federal spending that has increased each year, in spite of the tremendous pressures on the budget. However, the capacity of academic medicine to spend that money has increased at a faster rate than the research dollars, which had led to a relative under-supply of research dollars.

One issue is the size of the research enterprise and whether all academic health centers should try to compete in this realm. In fact, the market somewhat corrects for size. Another issue is whether clinicians who are essentially doing full-time research should be paid at a market-competitive salary.

The second mission is education. Nationally, we're faced with a paradox. Surveys of practicing clinicians in community medicine or private practice show that about 40% of doctors indicate that they would not go to medical school if they had the choice to do so again, and they are discouraging their sons, daughters, and colleagues about medical school. Yet we are witnessing the largest number of medical school applicants in history.

How do we reconcile these two phenomena? Students hear the message. However, they look at their colleagues trying to enter law and business and see that things are tough in these areas as well. Perhaps they have seen some unemployed lawyers driving taxis. As yet in the United States, there are no unemployed doctors, but if we keep training 24,000 residents per year, there may be some soon.

The market for education is still very good. The tension I see in the educational product is the conflict between the internal market, defined as what the academic medical center needs to satisfy its patient care activities, and the external market. One reason the market is not working as well is that medical students are buffered and see only the internal market.

A paper by Don Kassebaum in *Academic Medicine* last year showed the profiles of the outputs of generalist physicians among the different academic medical centers. Students enter medical centers with roughly the same goals, and about half of them are interested in being generalists. When they graduate from medical school A, only 5% of them may be generalists, compared to 50% of graduates from medical school B.

All graduates are facing the same external market, but those signals are blunted by faculty attitudes. The issue for academic medical centers is that if someone else pays for the product, and right now it is mainly government, what is your product responsibility? It doesn't make sense to contend that when someone buys something and asks for a product, that is regulation. I would call that prudent purchasing. If you turn to business to finance the GME and you have an all-payers system, it is unrealistic to say there will be no accountability for the products of that pool.

Academic medicine has to understand that the reason that school teachers and plumbers are paying tax monies to subsidize resident training is that they see this as a public good. Once something is being paid for by the public as a public good, it is unlikely that the profession will be able to determine the allocation of that good. That may not seem fair, but that is the way things work.

A real concern regarding education is the tuition cost and how that affects selection of students and their perception of careers. Medical school education is still a good investment, but the tuition in some institutions is as high as $30,000 per year for tuition only. I am concerned that as times get harder, academic medical centers will look to revenues from tuition when it is a seller's market and be tempted to raise tuition.

The research and educational missions are more attractive reasons for tax payers to help subsidize academic medicine than patient care. The academic patient care health delivery system, even though it is responsible for cross-subsidization, can be more difficult to defend. Of course, people want high-tech care when they can get it, but academia has done so well at training doctors to go into community hospitals that there are relatively few instances where high quality patient care can only be purchased at an academic center.

Clearly, there has been a tremendous growth in recent years of the clinical side of academic health science centers. It is assumed that most activities in the academic health science center enterprise depend upon clinical dollars, but it costs a lot of money to run those clinical programs, as well.

I am concerned about the capacity of academic health science centers to be competitive in the clinical arena under managed care, because of the culture of practice in academic medical centers where the sin of omission is far greater than the sin of commission, and the unspoken rule is, "Thou shalt not miss a case."

This is antithetical to the way that medicine is practiced in managed care. It is going to require a tremendous effort to develop the understanding of the faculty and to re-channel the clinical mission and the clinical culture.

I am confident that academic medicine will continue to survive, but it is unclear in what form, in particular, in regard to patient care entities. I suspect we will see even a greater divergence in the kinds of arrangements that are made locally and nationally than exist now.

*The Academic Health Center and Health
Care Reform,* edited by R. Snyderman,
M.C. Rogers, and V.Y. Saito.
Raven Press, Ltd., New York © 1995.

Toward Comprehensive Care

Daniel C. Tosteson, M.D.

Why aren't the NIH and Academic Health Centers (AHCs) revered in this culture? Why even raise the question that academic health centers might be considered irrelevant?

Several reasons come to mind. In a culture deeply beset with a rise of crime, violence, and ethnic conflict, one might wonder whether AHCs are addressing the **principal** problems of the society. Also, one might wonder why there is increased interest in alternative forms of medicine. Traditional medicine is accused of de-personalizing medical care and of promoting science-based medicine that does not take into account the personal nature of illness.

There is reason to believe that the science-based modern culture is poorly understood by the great majority of citizens in this country. Too often, they feel manipulated rather than helped by the discoveries being made in academic health centers.

It will be difficult to change without money, and money from traditional sources is becoming harder to find. On every front—direct income for education, research grant support, reimbursement for the delivery of clinical services by our faculties—we are facing the prospect of less money and less flexible money.

Economic necessity will drive us to invent new models for the synthesis of patient care, research, and education in the academic health centers of the future. A central effort will be redefining the interface between the traditional core academic enterprise and patient care.

Directions for change include more emphasis on ambulatory settings, primary care, the design and operation of multi-specialty clinics, and more attention to outcomes research. Research and education on disease prevention and public health education to produce more healthful behavior deserve broader effort.

This process of change is a long, evolutionary process that will be resolved over many years. Central to the resolution is the behavior of the physicians and health professionals who make up our faculties and our student bodies.

In the future, the most striking change in services provided by the academic health center will not be just away from tertiary, quaternary, rare disease care toward primary care, but rather toward comprehensive care. Only through providing comprehensive care in our academic health center will we be able to have the education and research environment appropriate for designing models for the health care of the future.

It is important that we not take on more than we can manage. We are not the entire health care system. We are the innovators of health care, and we should be approaching our work as model builders, not as operators of the national health care system.

The current circumstances provide unprecedented opportunities to improve the health of the American people. This is true in the molecular and cell biology laboratories and in clinical research, where discoveries made in those laboratories are employed in patients. There is plenty of room for improving the quality of outcomes research, actually developing measures of effectiveness of care. For all of these reasons, we should be speaking hopefully, not anxiously, as we participate in this great debate.

The Academic Health Center and Health
Care Reform, edited by R. Snyderman,
M.C. Rogers, and V.Y. Saito.
Raven Press, Ltd., New York © 1995.

Discussion

Professor Reinhardt: One had to concede that if the government pays for all of residency training and is the single buyer, then obviously the government has some right to determine what they buy. But should you allow institutions or even young physicians to develop a private market for residency training? People like myself would be quite comfortable with this approach and call it prudent purchasing, as long as it allowed some other market to exist where preferences on both sides could be expressed.

The state of New Jersey funds Rutgers, but it does not dictate what majors they offer. In Germany, however, the government funds the university and does dictate. They call it *numerus clausus.* You can have public funding like Rutgers and not have this dictation, whereas you do have it with the German model. This raises the discussion to whether government should be the only funder for this activity.

Dr. Pardes: Perhaps people might get the same kind of clinical care in multiple settings. But how do we preserve the notion of a critical mass in a given area of clinical research or clinical technology advance, which comes by having an academic health center with a sufficient group of students, teachers, clinicians, and academics who have a lot to do with advancing the field clinically?

If one were to develop a system in which the academic health centers were trimmed dramatically, in number or in size, would we be losing something in our ability to produce major advances in the technology that clinicians would have to help patients?

Different schools produce different percentages of primary care providers, and there is a tremendous amount of self-selection going on. It is likely that many students who want to go into the specialties or academic or research careers select the centers they attend.

One cannot say, if the turnout from a given school is less than from some other school, it is simply a function of environment. It has something to do with the population that chooses that particular school.

Dr. Schroeder: The general sense of both private and public purchasers of graduate medical education today is that there may be an over-supply of total numbers. There almost certainly is an over-supply of specialists. There probably is an under-supply of generalists, although that is not as clear. And the generalist market is now partially being cleared in the HMOs by nurse practitioners and PAs. A recent study showed that 40% of the urgent visits in one community health plan are to nurse practitioners.

My concern is that if this market does not get translated well to medical students, the current over-supply of physicians may start eating into medical school capacity if physicians void the generalist market and leave it to non-physicians. The policy of, "It is someone else's problem, not ours," could be quite foolish in the long run for academic medical centers.

Regarding Dr. Pardes' comments, I do not know the right clinical size for the innovation you discussed. Clearly, a critical mass is necessary, but I suspect it varies from one medical center to the other. I agree that a real danger of downsizing is that some of the innovation will be destroyed. It is not clear whether the size is right now. Maybe we are too small, and if so, we fall into that area of trade-offs.

The theory that the differences in expression of student generalist preference is a selection bias is not borne out by the paper I referred to, because it shows homogeneity in the expressed preferences of students as they enter medical school, while generalist preferences get selectively extinguished at different medical schools, more at some than at others.

Schools that have departments of family medicine are better able to nurture those preferences. In general, schools that have a more active research enterprise tend to extinguish generalism, but that is not exclusively true. I believe that UCSF and the University of Washington, which are in the top 10 in NIH funding, also are in the top 10 in producing generalists.

Dr. Tosteson: So long as we continue to have the current delta between the number of United States graduates and the number of PGY1 slots, there will be a suction of physicians worldwide, which makes our discussions of manpower planning ridiculous. Every year several thousand doctors are added to the systems that have been produced by educational systems over which we have no influence at all.

Another point which I believe has been under-emphasized is the other pole of what most of us would accept as the determinants of the great debate. Cost containment, we've talked about ad nauseam, but no one has mentioned access and security. And one very important traditional and continuing responsibility of academic health centers is to be alert to the needs of the underserved.

Mr. McMahon: Why do the academic health centers need to put themselves in the hands of an insurance company? Why can't we develop an integrated plan ourselves? Within the university there are other kinds of skills—actuarial, environmental, epidemiological. This should be our direction over time, although it will co-exist with fee-for-service.

Why can't we deal with the people much more intelligently than the insurance companies have proven that they can, or even than U.S. Health Care and Well Point have been able to do?

Mr. James A. Lane: The difference is that we have patients and members and HMOs and insurers have members and they also have patients, but they get those members from insurance companies and employers.

If you were to try to replicate what we have, for example, which we started from scratch and built a whole delivery system, you would have to recruit 1 million members for a 1,000-bed medical center.

The fundamental problem is this cannot be accomplished overnight. As was suggested, in the process, you may alienate people who will cut you off from many potential patients.

Dr. Mulvihill: Let us assume they could do that. Another problem is that not many academic health centers would be willing or able to take the risk. Are you willing to take the financial risk associated with insuring the health of a given population?

Secondly, are you able and willing to take the risk of being the least-expensive provider, or one of two or three least expensive? You have quality and you have the name of the university, therefore allowing you to attract and retain those patients.

Moderator Relman: That raises some very interesting questions. Is it practical or desirable for academic health centers to form their own HMO, their own managed care plan? Are there limitations on the size? What should be the strategy?

Dr. Langfitt: Most academic health centers are large, distinguished organizations with very fine reputations within their regions, and they do not, by virtue of what they do, really understand what it means to insure lives and to insure health care. It is obviously a very complicated business with its own experience and traditions.

There might be an opportunity for the academic health center to link up with a distinguished insurer—companies that have a long tradition of being financially sound—and to see whether it is possible to pair an academic health center with a major insurer.

Dr. Robinson: I would tell any academic health center that is putting together a network that one needs to take a very careful look at whom one is excluding. You may run the risk of subjecting your institution to just about as much risk as if you did not put together that network.

I can see that in our own environment every day—intensely competitive, everyone wishing to partner up with everyone else, and as you partner, someone is left out.

Mr. Gary A. Mecklenburg: The nation's teaching hospitals have been handled quite well in recent years, despite all the difficulties that exist. I believe, however, that if the academic medical center and teaching hospital are going to be in the competitive marketplace, they have to be competitive.

For example, 10 years ago my hospital was the most expensive hospital in Chicago. Today, it is the least expensive of any major teaching hospital. Our length of stay is lower than most hospitals, or comparable to that of many other hospitals.

I had to sign a contract last year for cardiovascular services that was 50% of my usual and customary charges. I believe this is inescapable.

Many fine community hospitals are performing the same services that we do in our academic medical centers much less expensively, using the people that we have trained and the technology we have transferred. But the reality is that every time I've examined the three academic medical center hospitals I have helped manage, 70% of what is offered in an academic medical center is the same as what is offered by community hospitals, and they are doing it a lot less expensively. We have to learn from that and be competitive, if we are going to continue to be in the marketplace.

Alternatively, as we see in the better developed marketplaces, our academic medical center hospitals will be low-volume, high-specialty places. I chuckle at the idea of making these centers for-profit, stock-issuing corporations. I am not sure who would buy them.

Dr. Martin: As a member of a public institution, I would like to respond to the issue that taxpayers expect a public university to deliver the goods in terms of the primary versus specialty care interests. In California, we have faced legislation for the past 3 years that would mandate 50% of residency positions in primary care, with the incentive being that failure to do so will result in the elimination of the money allocated for residency training. This has happened despite the fact that UCSF's budget from the state is only 13% of our total budget.

At a time when the California economy is failing and student fees are rising, for the past 2 years the legislators have dipped into hospital revenues and taken money away from the positive bottom lines to subsidize other things. You can imagine how discouraging that is to effective and skilled hospital administrators who are working very hard to create revenue for the next year.

Dr. Biles: We now have something on the order of 24,000 residents, compared to the number of approximately 17,000 graduates. Thus, we are up to almost 140% of first-year residents. We are importing large numbers of international graduates, and the number continues to increase at about 4% a year.

There's been no indication here of a market response, or else the market is different. The market is more hospital administrators and people working essentially 40 hours a week at fairly modest pay.

The administration's bill doesn't specify a number, but the Rockefeller-Waxman bill suggests the number ought to be something on the order of 110% of United States graduates. That would phase down the total number of physicians and, of course, this phasing down would occur on the specialty and the subspecialty side of the equation over a period of something like 10 years.

The Academic Health Center and Health
Care Reform, edited by R. Snyderman,
M.C. Rogers, and V.Y. Saito.
Raven Press, Ltd., New York © 1995.

Responses

Arthur Garson, Jr., M.D., M.P.H.: I challenge the concept that all that the clinical functions of academic health centers can be reproduced outside. Perhaps this is possible for 30% to 40% of what we do. However, at our institution we analyzed one of our services to try to transfer the general patients to a general hospital. After thorough consultation, we decided about 5% of our general patients could be transferred to a general hospital.

I question the notion that we are taking care of the same patient. I am not sure whether risk adjustment is going to take care of that.

I'm concerned about a critical mass of patient care, not just a critical mass of research. Critical mass of patients involves doctors such as the three pediatric rheumatologists referred to previously. We don't even need three. But how do we merge and regionalize with other services?

We've made an attempt in cardiology to merge with the UNC Pediatric Cardiology Division for 2 years, and that is about as easy as merging basketball teams from two institutions. Unfortunately, there is nothing in any legislation that promotes regionalization or provides incentive to get together other than the market.

William New, Jr., M.D., Ph.D.: I am the only representative from the world of small-business, high-tech, venture-capital-fueled Silicon Valley innovation.

Today, academic centers are filled with well-trained, bright people, knowledgeable workers interested in research and innovation, who want to work with smart people and the latest and best equipment. They don't want to worry about their financial futures. They certainly have great needs for autonomy. They want time for inspiration.

They are in a world that is flooded with international graduates and are finding themselves attracted away from the academic sector over to the private sector, frankly to make more money, to have better access to research facilities, and to achieve their dreams. I'm not talking about medicine. I'm talking about engineering and business schools, which represent the other professional schools on the campus. These schools are relatively successful. Perhaps we should consider what they have done to attract these students and how they are succeeding, because they have encountered many of the issues discussed at this conference.

They, too, have the three missions of teaching, research and practice. The interesting thing is they do teaching and research, but unlike medicine, they don't practice on the campus. We're following a 19th-century model of appren-

56

ticeship by having our practice in the hospital right here on the campus. The business school doesn't run businesses on the campus. The engineering school doesn't run manufacturing lines. So, I wonder if we're doing the wrong thing.

Are the missions of the AHC relevant to society? The teaching, absolutely; the research, partially. I would submit that the research that is done outside of industry, and I would pick engineering as an example, outstrips that which is done in academia. It is the same phenomenon we are starting to see in medicine and practice. Should we have practice in hospitals on campus? Frankly, that is doubtful. It is not the skill setting.

Why and how would these missions change? The reason we are changing is the current environment of short-term economics. University medical centers think in terms of long-term, not short-term economics. We are hopelessly mismatched for the task at hand.

What do we do that is unique? We're the Keeper of the Flame! We are the folks who are going to pass it on to the next generation and that, in fact, should be the service that we provide—the ideas, thoughts, the model builders, the innovation.

What should we not be doing? We should not be doing anything that we are not good at. I do not believe we should be running hospitals or raising capital or trying to make a profit, though of course we would never use such Philistine terms. We would call it retained surplus.

We appear to be involved in a paradigm shift. Academic health centers started the current paradigm in the early 1950s with NIH and into the 1960s with Medicare. In the prewar era, we ran medical centers in a completely different way.

In the last generation, American medical centers have become the priesthood in the same way that the Anglican Church, the Church of England, has faded from its 19th-century prominence. It is still around, but appears to be nonexistent.

I would urge that we not fall into the same model as the NIH, with the research model funding everything from the government. We should change that and develop a new model.

I do not believe we can evolve out of this market. My colleague pointed out the obvious, i.e., it would take 1 million insured lives to run a medical center today. It cannot be done.

Robert G. Petersdorf, M.D.: We have become too large, and we have to cut down the system. Nine years ago we had 72,000 residents; we now have 102,000. We had 13,000 FMGs 9 years ago, and we now have 23,000. We are still part of the biggest bull market that the world has ever seen. The best we can say about the latest residency match is that some specialties did not increase in size.

I suggested 9 years ago that we cut the house staff first and the medical school second. I have now come to the conclusion that the entire academic apparatus is too large. The residency programs are too large. We have too many medical students, but it is politically very difficult to cut medical school class sizes in public schools when there are many more applicants than ever before.

Some recent data showed that the number of Ph.D.s and postdoctoral students in biomedical science is far too great. Young people seem to recognize this. They have composed a letter from the Society for Young Scientists to Harold Varmus, the NIH director, saying, "We cannot get any jobs."

Not only can't they get any jobs, they also remain in Ph.D. and postdoctoral programs for years on end because they can't find anything else to do. All of this reinforces the thesis that the size of the entire academic establishment is too large.

The academic establishment is also terribly expensive. That is not to say that we do not produce, under certain circumstances, outstanding quality medical care. A recent article in *Newsweek* reported that a number of doctors in the United States make $1 million each year; drug company executives and hospital administrators in this country get paid a lot more than in the rest of the world. Drugs are more expensive, hospitals are more expensive, and almost everything having to do with health care is more expensive.

Suppose one simply cut 20% off the bill. We could then cope much more readily with some of the difficult issues, because cost control is at the bottom of the gyrations that are going on in the system.

We have to look at the expenses inherent in health care. The actuarial studies of the Health Security Act have explored the expense side of the ledger in depth and agree that costs are too high.

I agree with Dr. New that we do not fit into the mold of the managed care system. The *modus operandi* of department chairmen and deans does not fit the managed care culture. If we're going to compete with the managed care culture, we are going to have to do things differently. On the other hand, I am not sure that we want to do them differently or, indeed, that we should do them differently.

The Academic Health Center and Health Care Reform, edited by R. Snyderman, M.C. Rogers, and V.Y. Saito. Raven Press, Ltd., New York © 1995.

General Discussion

Dr. Pardes: I would like to ask Dr. New to expand on his provocative comments regarding the keepers of the flame and the model builders. Where will those models be built and where will the flames be kept if we dispose ourselves of academic hospitals? I would also like him to expand on what could replace the NIH in support of the basic biomedical research.

Dr. New: Dr. Tosteson's organization tries not to run very many hospitals and my belief is that MIT doesn't try to run very many manufacturing plants. The fact that hospitals are not under our direct control does not make us any less able to practice our craft. I am not saying we should not practice our craft. What I am saying is that we should not be in the hospital business.

In my view, the NIH has served a useful social purpose, probably modeled much after the Manhattan Project, but it has become way too big. We have, in fact, created a whole culture that has produced this over-supply of Ph.D.s who work for the government indirectly.

I believe there should be some national center of excellence, but I think we should scale down the NIH and get back to excellence. It is a question of scale, not excellence.

Dr. Tosteson: Several people have talked about the incompatibility of managed care and the academic cultures. It is worth noting that there are some modest exceptions to that general rule.

Harvard has an affiliated HMO, the Harvard Community Health Plan, which now is the locus for an academic department, the Department of Ambulatory Care and Prevention, in which substantial residency training and medical student training takes place. Of course there is some friction, but many constructive activities go on as well.

Dr. Langfitt: The issue we are discussing appears to be whether it is feasible and, if so, desirable for there to be a separation of functions within the academic medical center.

The vertically integrated system that most people feel will be necessary for most academic health centers to compete for patients and patient revenues is a justified system that is needed to educate our medical students and to train our residents in the most appropriate kind of ways.

Many of us are proud that so much of clinical education tends to take place on the hospital floors in an organ-based, disease-specific, price-oriented kind of medicine. Those students and trainees end up out in office practices doing various kinds of medical practice.

This kind of system provides the full range of opportunities for education and training for residents and students. This is the same kind of a vertically integrated system that is optimal for patient care clinical research, including medical trials, and, particularly, outcomes research and outcomes management.

Dr. Waller: We don't see another alternative to competing. We have all been competing for years and will do so far into the future. There does not appear to be a "cookie cutter" approach to the competitive strategy of the future. For us, it has included in the past decade: the development of an IPA model prepaid health plan in southeast Minnesota, managed care contracts, management contracts, integration with hospitals, affiliations with other physicians, new relationships with industry, mergers with small, medium and large clinics, and the development of Mayo Group Practices in Arizona and Florida. There is a long list of options for the coming decade to add to these initiatives.

Dr. Petersdorf: I don't think we should attempt to run these centers with our faculties providing the primary care. I was the second Visiting Professor at the Harvard Community Health Plan. They have a different culture that taught me a lot, and I found most of the things they do entirely admirable.

When I was Dean at San Diego we had a tough time with our affiliation with Kaiser of Southern California, particularly when it came to selling our medical students to that HMO for primary care training. Kaiser did not mind the residents and they particularly liked the residents in neurosurgery. But they certainly did not like the students, because the students interfered with their productivity. Unfortunately, that is true in a lot of HMOs in today's world.

The relationships we are forging between academic medical centers and managed care organizations represent a new world for us. We should not jump right into the middle of it, at least as primary operators of an HMO, because we are more likely not to succeed than to succeed.

Dr. Pardes: We have been cautioned that because academic health centers will be seeking multiple vendors to invest in or to make arrangements with, you put yourself at risk if you develop your own managed care system in competition with other vendors.

There are any number of instances in which joint administration of medical school and the hospital work very well. The Mount Sinai Medical Center in New York is one example.

One useful question for this group is to discuss the question of split versus unified administration between hospitals and medical schools.

The notion that the NIH is too big because there are too many Ph.D.s doesn't seem logical. One could argue that perhaps we have too many applicants for NIH grants and perhaps we have an over-supply of young people coming through our research programs, but I do not agree that the NIH is too big. I would question whether it is big enough in terms of research dollars.

The federal labs program accounts for approximately 60% of the federal science budget. That amount is much greater than the number of dollars being put into biomedical research. I think the NIH has been a very successful investment, and I would hope it would be sustained even if we decided that we should train fewer Ph.D.s.

Dr. Bruce J. Sams: I realize that it will be difficult for academic centers to develop their own managed care program, and possibly expensive. However, having watched the competitive market at work and observing that the power lies with the owner in such a system, I can predict that AHCs that do not have control will eventually be unhappy as participants in someone else's system.

The strongest systems will manage and control an integrated system oriented toward patient care, teaching, and research. It must have full support and commitment from its members, who must feel that their efforts are producing results which they value— that is, they are not working for someone else or someone else's goals.

Dr. Snyderman: It is clear that we need to educate our students in an ambulatory care environment. It is becoming increasingly difficult to do so unless we have the option of having a firmer linkage with the ambulatory care clinics outside of our medical center. In a place like Duke, our focus is on specialty clinics and a specialty-oriented hospital.

Physicians who are not part of our faculty are finding it increasingly difficult to provide our learners with medical education, and this is felt more in California than it is here. Physicians affiliated with other plans are saying, "How can we afford to take your students on, because the people who are paying us are not going to pay us to do that?" To some degree we need to redevelop the system to be able to educate the students.

Steven Schroeder discussed the extinction of medical students' desire for a general practice as they go through medical school. I can confirm that. When we poll entering Duke University students on their desire to go into general practice, between 60% and 70% indicate interest in some profession related to general practice. That interest is maintained until somewhere around the third year, when there is a shift toward going into the specialties. Part of the reason for that may be the selection of our students, but I suspect this is a minor component.

Practicing primary care physicians seem to be different in terms of motivating factors and sources of self-esteem compared to the usual Duke student at the time of graduation. The education at Duke Hospital drives a lot of people to specialty care because that is what they see.

The alternative to our developing a primary care network is to be totally dependent on an insurer getting 32% of the health care dollar before they really start dealing with us. If that happens, I believe that we may jeopardize our entire system.

The external network in which we engage in managed care probably ought not to be the same faculty as we have in the academic medical center. We need to develop an external network that is either run by us or run in a joint venture in which we have substantial control of our services. Our health services need to be closer to the consumer to assure the viability of the medical center core by allowing some of the front-end margin that one gets with capitated managed care to flow back into the system.

I agree that we ought not to do it ourselves, but I think we need to be intimately involved with a partner who will not expunge all the margin before it gets to us and freeze us out of the educational network.

Dr. Robinson: Although networking has many advantages, it makes the decision process difficult, because networking requires choosing sides, and it potentially requires sharing responsibility for decision-making over university programs with others who have not heretofore shared in those things.

Size is another concern. I am amazed every time I come back to Duke about how many more buildings have been added and the same statement might be applied to our institution. All of our centers continue to act as if we are infinitely expansible.

Dr. Tosteson: My sense is that our core mission is bench-to-bedside research, the continuum of education, and truly innovative care, and we should keep those in front of us as we participate in these discussions. We should encourage our clinical faculties to organize their practices with emphasis on this core mission.

Dr. Waller: The discussions on downsizing bring to mind that size is one thing and profile is another. One of the major questions for us will be the size and profile of our faculty as we look to the future.

We are increasingly convinced that vertically integrated systems really do save money in terms of reducing the expense base for a practice. In addition, for us, inpatient care is not the core business.

Dr. Biles: What are teaching costs in a world with universal health insurance coverage? If every patient, both inpatient and outpatient, has health insurance and pays at essentially mainstream rates, what are the residual additional costs of teaching institutions?

Plans now pay a 20% to 30% differential for teaching hospitals. The assumption discussed here is that future plans will pay some lesser amount—5% to 10%. Can the centers generate additional savings on the order of 5% to 10%?

Dr. Rabkin: Indeed, there are savings to be accrued at academic health centers, and we had better do our best to achieve them. The fact that $9.6 billion is a lot of money is not terribly meaningful if, in fact, today's actual amount paid projects to something like $21 to $24 billion.

Perhaps more important is the assumption that this is based on universal health care. What if universal health care is not enacted and we still have the uninsured? Even if there is universal health care, we have the aliens and people who are uncovered.

All of us are waiting for the other shoe to drop. The private payer today who has a contract for $1 and whose contract will end in 2 years . . . let's say Medicaid is paying hospitals at 80 cents . . . we know that the private payer will start out negotiating the next contract opening at 72 cents. We are headed for a big dip from the private sector as well.

Dr. Pardes: When one describes the pools of money coming through the proposed Health Security Act, we should note whether there has been some positive response from the administration recognizing what many of us have argued for—a medical school stream of money independent of the hospital monies. We are trying to get reasonable estimates of that, but a rough range would be about $1.5 billion.

Dr. Waller: Could we hear more about how these dollars might be distributed?

Dr. Biles: The direct medical education funds in the amount of $5.8 billion would be paid out on a per-resident amount, which is a national average adjusted for wages and other factors. Those payments under Medicare have historically been substantially higher than the national average. In New York and some of the hospitals in Boston, there have been some questions about a phase-in from current levels to a per-resident amount.

Dr. Waller: Would that per-resident amount include residents in ambulatory settings as well?

Dr. Biles: These monies go on the training side now, rather than directly to the hospitals.

Dr. Petersdorf: We would like to have the funds funneled to an entity that applies on behalf of programs. It could be a hospital; a medical school; an HMO; or a group practice, if that is the way the entity wanted to set it up. We are not directive about that, but the entity needs to be accountable and needs to be relatively smaller than the 4,000 training programs which we now have.

Dr. Biles: On the indirect side, which is on the hospital side, $3.8 billion would flow to the hospitals, and each individual hospital would essentially get its share based on the current Medicare rate, which is the resident-per-bed ratio. Institutions with many more residents per bed get the bulk of the money times essentially the size of the hospital, which would be measured by inpatient and perhaps outpatient revenues.

Dr. Pardes: I want to underline that one of the other things the AAMC is advocating is the possible consortium of medical schools and hospitals that would be the recipient of those GME monies.

Dr. Rabkin: If you're paying out on the basis of national averages, then hospitals in Boston and New York, for a variety of reasons, will be paid relatively less than their actual costs, but is it implied that the others whose actual costs are even lower will receive the national average?

Dr. Biles: The best data we have is Medicare dated 1984, trended forward. We know that in 1984, hospitals had very different practices.

Some of them, particularly in New York City, put a lot of attending physician costs on the hospital side, and so those hospitals today have high hospital inpatient per-resident amounts. On the other hand, hospitals, particularly in Texas, were billing on the outpatient side, and since they were supposed to refrain from double billing, they actually put very little money on the inpatient or hospital costs.

To go back to universal coverage, it is an issue that the committees are monitoring. The discussion tends to focus on transition. If we have universal coverage, then the hospitals which now have their attending costs billed on the inpatient side, will likely set up faculty practice plans like the other hospitals around the country. Therefore, to continue to pay them large amounts on the inpatient side poses the question of double payment.

The approach is to try to start where people are today, but over time to presume there will be a transition to a more nationally uniform pattern.

Moderator Relman: In principle, I hear no argument against the proposition that the costs of education of residents is a legitimate charge against the third-party payers. No one has a better proposal for meeting that expense.

Dr. Mulvihill: For 50% to 60% of certain specialty residency positions in dentistry, the cost is up to $20,000 to $25,000 a year in tuition for the opportunity.

Moderator Relman: Why not charge residents tuition for going into a specialty after they complete their 3 years of basic training?

Dr. Langfitt: You could just split it between the faculty and the residents, because the faculty get most of the benefit out of it in terms of work they do not have to do.

Dr. Pardes: My impression is that residents provide a tremendous amount of clinical care that is valued by the reimbursement system. They are, in a sense, paying off their tuition by performing clinical care.

Also, these medical students are now in debt up to $75,000 to $100,000, and this would be another $100,000 in debt for them. Given the fact that we are discussing a likely reworking of the reimbursement system for different specialties, those salaries will come down and this loads prohibitive costs on them.

Professor Reinhardt: You can compare the level of education of someone with an M.D. with that of a young lawyer starting out and then compare salary level. Physicians are already paying tuition relative to the value added, if you could calculate the value added. The hospitals probably pay them no more than value added minus what it costs to train them.

Dr. Schroeder: I believe there is a paper in press in *The New England Journal of Medicine* that looks at opportunity costs and finds that for specialty physicians, for lawyers, and for business people, stratified for class standing and GPAs, there is a return on equity for training. Under current market conditions, there is not such a return for generalist physicians.

Dr. Rabkin: When you look at further specialty training beyond residency, that is, specialty fellowships, often those salaries are half of what the fellows were earning as residents. There is an economic toll for specialty training.

Dr. Langfitt: It gets back to this issue of why we have 7,000 more residency positions than we have graduates from American medical schools, and why the percentages of numbers increased by 30% in the past 9 years. Costs go up to 72%, 30% or 40% for your total number of residencies.

The main need for residents is to provide service. This process allows the faculty and staff to reduce their work load in terms of what residents do. We should be rethinking why we have so many residents as well as who pays for it.

Dr. Snyderman: An obvious target for right-sizing or expense reduction within the medical center and the hospital is the size of graduate medical education and is an area we have just begun to look at. I can tell you it is not obvious whether you actually save money when you cut physicians because of their ability to generate clinical revenues.

At Duke, and I suspect at other places, we are paying the salaries, particularly of the fellows, out of the practice plans. One of the largest areas of cross-subsidization is to pay for fellows, or some of the residents that have been in residency beyond the 4 years.

Mr. McMahon: You all are thinking in terms of the continuation of the current dollar "fee-for-service" end of the practice plan. What if you were paid on a capitation basis, at least for some of the patients, or that you begin to think in capitation terms. You perceive the resident a little differently. All of a sudden, he or she may be another pair of hands at a much lower cost and, compared to the community hospital and community physician sector, a much lower-cost provider of a range of care.

If you do not consider these dual terms of how the money is going to start to flow, then some of you will solve the residency question in the fee-for-service setting at the same time that others of you are looking toward the capitation setting.

Dr. Waller: A real problem is related to penalties for efficient markets. In Olmsted County, Minnesota, if we were to develop a Medicare HMO in 1994 and have it capitated on a per-member, per-month basis and try to train residents, we would be paid $363 per member, per month, which is down to 0.5% in 1993. In Los Angeles, payment would be $531 per month, up 15%; in Dade County, Florida, $574 per month, up 20%; in Kings County, New York, $610 per month, up 84%.

The hospital wage index in Olmsted County was reduced 9% in 1993! The manner in which dollars are distributed now is clearly in need of revision.

Dr. Pardes: I wonder what your reactions would be to the proposition that it is in the interests of the health of the academic health centers that some federal legislation be passed and that we are at greatest risk if there is no legislation.

A corollary to that would be, if so, what do you want in the legislation, and what changes would be to the advantage of the academic health center?

A second question is, What common advice or prescription can you give to academic health centers? Are there common principles or steps we can take that make sense for the majority of academic health centers?

Dr. Schroeder: Dr. Pardes, why do you think it is in their best interests to have the bill passed?

Dr. Pardes: It may take a long time in getting there, but I take it as a right principle that there be total coverage in this country. I think total coverage will be to the benefit of the academic health centers. To do something to equalize the capacity of people to purchase health care is both a right policy and also right for the academic health centers.

The academic health centers are going to need the kind of additional help that the Health Security Act would seem to be moving toward providing, and that would not be available if you simply had the forces of managed care.

Dr. Rogers: In one way it would simplify the environment, because it would remove the need to be competitive from the academic health center, and to that extent, it would deal with a number of issues about our mission.

Everything comes at a price, and the price would be our ultimate dependence on decisions made by the government with which we would not be comfortable. It is a simplistic answer, but the ultimate consequences are dependent on forces we cannot see fully over a long period of time.

Mr. Mecklenburg: Under an all-payer system, the assumption is that everyone is going to get paid the same, but then we are going to get paid more. I'm not sure that you can count on that.

Are we going to be treated differently? I'm not sure that we are going to be treated differently under an all-payer system or under market forces.

The battle we are fighting right now is that IME stands out as a separate payment, and it has consistently been attacked over a long period of time. Can the teaching hospital or academic health center continue to justify its difference to the satisfaction of regulators, government officials, and the marketplace?

Moderator Relman: I attended a meeting of the Ontario Medical Association when the Ministry of Health was announcing to the Association members that tax revenues that year in Ontario reflecting the continued recession or depression there, were lower than anticipated, and, therefore, the Ministry of Health could not meet its promise made the previous year to negotiate a new fee schedule with the Ontario doctors beginning with cost-of-living. The promise they had made was that, "We would start negotiations with a cost-of-living, across-the-board increase and then see where we would go from there."

The Deputy Minister of Health said that he was very sorry, but that the funds simply were not available. Not only were they not going to give a cost-of-living, across-the-board increase and negotiate, there would be no collective bargaining, and they were going to start with a 7% cut across-the-board.

After that, one of the leaders of the Ontario Medical Association said to me, "You see what happens when a tax-supported system depends on general revenues. If you Americans ever go to a tax-supported system, never have it come from general revenues but have it be earmarked so the taxes can only be spent on health care."

I do not believe anybody would argue that if you had to depend on the legislative process every year for what you were paid that it would be an unstable, unreliable arrangement.

Dr. Martin: Welcome to California. That's exactly what we are doing. We had a 5% across-the-board cut.

Moderator Relman: Could that be avoided by having an earmarked tax which could only be spent on health care and having a quasi-public agency like a Federal Reserve Board, which was public and private, that decided how that money was going to be spent? Would that be any better, or are we concluding that there is simply no way that the United States' health care system can be supported by taxes without having the system break down?

Dr. New: Every time we have had an airplane ticket in the last 20 years we have been paying into an airport fund. For all intents and purposes, that fund is impounded. It is instructed to invest its money in the federal treasuries so that, in essence, much like you are experiencing with somebody in the government going into your hospital funds, the federal government can go into the impounded funds.

The reality of that is the political will is the political will is the political will!

We are seeking some way that the M.D. and the academic health center can rise above the fray. It is not possible, unfortunately, and we have to figure out either how to avoid the problem, or be better at it than the next person.

Dr. Rogers: When we provide funds for graduate medical education, they start at $9 billion and they get up to $15 and $20 billion, beginning to approach the range of the farm subsidy.

How many people think that we would be able to protect politically how we fare relative to the power of the farmer to be protected if there was a bad crop? I am sure they would use our subsidy to give to the farmers. There are a lot more of them than there are of us.

Dr. Mulvihill: There are four possible considerations for tactics. First would be to inspire your faculty with your vision and your mission and your goals. Second, try to get your faculty practices to be more cohesive and less splintered.

Third, set up some good information systems, because these will be needed as we move further into managed care and increased competitiveness.

Finally, keep your eyes on your governors and your state legislators. They will have much to say under most federal health care reform proposals.

We concentrate all the time on what will happen at the federal level, and I think there will be a lot of room, at the governors' requests, at the state level.

Dr. Tosteson: It appears that we cannot afford to act as if there will be no legislation. We must be fully involved in helping to mold legislation so that it is beneficial to the country and consistent with our institutional goals.

There are many champions of cost containment and very few champions of quality. We have to stand strongly on that side, urging the legislators to realize that a learning health care system, one in which continuing education and practice are interwoven at the grass roots, is the road to quality. Although we have not implemented it adequately, it is a message that warrants repetition.

The other realm is the whole issue of providing care to the underserved and access to community service. We should be championing that from a political perspective, as well as from a moral and ethical perspective.

Dr. Anlyan: If we are discussing graduate medical education, let us not forget the Veterans Administration (VA). What is going to happen there is important to many of the academic medical centers.

The VA is an example of a single-payer system in the United States. It would seem to me that the VA is a few years behind in the quality of the care offered across the street at Duke. In many instances, the VA is subsidized by the academic medical center. Its global budget is in competition with everything else on the federal scene and it has to compete for its share of the pie.

Dr. Snyderman: Regarding whether we do better with legislation than without legislation, I have a comment. Up until recently, we were embedding two-thirds of our non-reimbursed academic costs in our clinical charges, and we were able to do so because of how we were paid. As of now, we can no longer do so. We are facing catastrophic changes that are going to force us to do several things.

One of them is to be as competitive and cost effective as possible in every area. When all is said and done, we cannot compete on any open marketplace, given the added cost of what we do.

Although I agree with everything that has been said about the vulnerability one has in relying on tax structures of any sort, I believe it is inevitable that society will have to pay for the added value that we bring to health care. Much of the benefit we provide is not achieved on the day that it is delivered, but is an ongoing process that improves quality over time. If we cannot make that argument convincing, it is our own fault.

In relating this to the farm subsidy, health care is equally valuable or more valuable to the economy than the farm subsidy. We comprise 15% of the GNP. Everyone has to rely on us for the quality of their health care. We have to be more articulate in making that case for subsidies for our education and research missions because I do not see any other choice, no matter how good we become.

The Academic Health Center and Health Care Reform, edited by R. Snyderman, M.C. Rogers, and V.Y. Saito. Raven Press, Ltd., New York © 1995.

Session III: How Will Health Care Delivery Systems for the AHC Change in an Era of Reform?

Overview

Mark C. Rogers, M.D., M.B.A., Moderator

Although it is generally assumed that we are going to be forming health networks or health systems, we have not really asked the question: Is the health system or the health network the answer to the problems confronting academic medical centers? How do we define the answer and how do we define success?

Even though I am charged with the responsibility of helping develop the health network at Duke University, I have some key reservations. One is that there is reason to believe that the health network will not replace existing clinical incomes.

At Duke, we transfer $100 to $150 million out of clinical income from the hospital and the clinical practice, either above the profit line in terms of cross-subsidization or below the profit line in terms of actually taking the profit and reinvesting it. To replace these resources from a health network at a 10% rate of return, we would need a $1.5 billion enterprise to run. We must also reserve some money for keeping that $1.5 billion enterprise operating next year, as well as have finances to invest in some new facilities. Soon we will need a $2 to $2.5 billion enterprise, using hundreds of thousands of patients to generate these resources.

Some of you come from cities of three, four, five, six, seven, eight million people. Some of us come from cities with 300,000 people. Regardless of size, putting together a health network of hundreds of thousands of members is a challenge, because in the place where there are eight million people, there are nine million health organizations. In a place with a 300,000 population, the health organization is spread out over several hundred miles. Even if the business is successful, this does not address how the faculty are affected in their academic missions by the geographic distribution. Nor does it address the change in composition of clinicians who are primary care versus specialists.

Presently, we have 40–50 specialists for every primary care doctor. If we use faculty for our network, we would have to add dozens and dozens of primary care doctors.

We have to ask the questions: Should we do it? How do we do it? Do we do it alone? Do we do it with a commercial strategic partner? Do we do it among a series of academic institutions?

It has been suggested that it would be reasonable for us to do it alone. After all, we have actuarial data, and we have all kinds of schools in the university to build a business. However, there are companies with billions of dollars in assets who claim that the insurance industry is an expertise in and of itself. They believe that it is easier for an insurance company to buy a primary care practice than it is for a primary care practice to learn the expertise of an insurance company.

That doesn't encompass the capitalization requirements of setting up a network. In our state, there is a nationally known organization which has targeted $100 million to invest in this region—$100 million that they're going to spend not on facilities, but on buying practices and advertising, signing up patients, signing up employees. That is $100 million that we do not have to spend.

As a result, there are valid reasons for us to analyze whether we do this alone, with a commercial strategic partner, or with an academic partner. Each has different organizational implications.

This is a simplistic model of the challenge that we have in putting together one of these organizations. We have physicians who provide tertiary care and very expensive facilities, perhaps in areas that are distributed to multiple hospitals and multiple clinics, multiple capital investments. Regardless of the choice, we are going to be faced with a faculty that wants to be buffered from decreasing incomes. We must expect that they will question each of us, because we will be investing tens of millions of dollars of what they see as their money in buying practices and information systems at a time of decreasing rates of reimbursement.

What competence do we have to do this? What organizations do we have to do this? Finally, do we have a culture that will promote business success?

We will hear this morning from a person in a for-profit company who is charged with competing with us, a person who does nothing but buy practices, whose boss can agree to buy a practice in 1 minute or agree to buy a group of practices for $25 or $30 or $40 million.

That individual can pay anything he wants for those practices. We are limited, as many of you will be, in bidding competitively for practices or for facilities. Because of our not-for-profit status, we are limited by law in what we can pay relative to market value. For-profit organizations are not limited in what they can invest, because they can buy market share to put us out of the running early in the game.

What organization develops the academic health network? Is it the university with which your academic medical center is involved? Is it the hospital? Is it the medical school? Is it the faculty practice? Is it a hybrid organization? Can you go into this business if you are a state school?

What number of people over what period of time can make business decisions for the academic network, and what number of trustees and administrators and chairpersons, and faculty need to be convinced in order to come to a decision?

We have real problems if we do not deal with all of our constituencies, but if we do deal with them, the time it takes represents an alternate set of problems.

Do we have effective control over our business decisions? If we have a commercial business partner, how does our organization work? Do we use the Columbia name? Do we use the Duke name? Do we use the Harvard name? If we do not, have we gotten full market value for what we have to offer?

Whose boards of directors sit down to allocate the expenses and allocate the profits? Is it the university, the department chairs, the hospital, the medical school?

When we discuss academic health centers reformatted to have health networks, we are discussing a hybrid that begins with a series of values that we share with the university on one hand and with the business world on the other hand. Those values we share with the university are commitments to education and research. The value we share with business is the desire to be profitable, albeit with the intention to reinvest our profits in research and education.

The challenge we face is the need to reconcile the conflicting organizational structures and values of these competing goals. We will not be successful in a practical fashion unless we have a better conceptual understanding of how to reconcile these conflicts.

The Academic Health Center and Health Care Reform, edited by R. Snyderman, M.C. Rogers, and V.Y. Saito. Raven Press, Ltd., New York © 1995.

The Need for Strategic Planning

William N. Kelley, M.D.

I will focus on the health services at the University of Pennsylvania and re-emphasize that our health services strategic planning is part of an overall strategic planning effort that involves our educational programs, research programs, as well as health services programs. It also has involved development, financial planning, and master-site facilities planning.

We have conducted this planning in parallel over the last four-and-a-half years I've been at Penn. Over the last year or so, we have brought the plans together and are well under way in implementation.

Our health services strategic plan led us to decide that we needed to focus on seven clinical program areas of emphasis: cancer, musculoskeletal diseases, neurosciences, transplant, cardiac diseases, women's health, and gastrointestinal disorders.

This effort led us to take a different approach at our distribution strategy for providing care that is not only on-site ambulatory care but off-site ambulatory care, involving both primary care and multispecialty satellites.

We have developed 150 or so principles that have to do with quality of service, what we call the principles of practice. How many times should the phone ring? When should the clinics and offices be open for appointments? How long should one have to wait for an appointment? How long should one look for a parking place?

The process also led us to conclude we needed a different approach to managed care and a different approach to hospital affiliations. Finally, it resulted in a strategic business plan for health services, and it led us to conclude that we needed to develop a health system.

Let me focus on the latter—the University of Pennsylvania Health System corporate organizational structure, as it was approved by the trustees on June 18, 1993. It involves the University of Pennsylvania Medical Center as it has stood in recent years. The Medical Center itself includes the School of Medicine, with its academic programs and its clinical practices, as well as the Hospital of the University of Pennsylvania, which remains the same in this new structure. In addition to the medical center, we have added the health care network with the following components:

- Physician network.
- Multiple off-site ambulatory care facilities.

- A different relationship with hospitals and other provider organizations.
- A managed care organization.
- A management services organization.

Based on our analysis of the region and our needs, both from an educational perspective as well as to provide a geographically distributed primary care network in the immediate Greater Philadelphia area, and based on extensive marketing research, we concluded that we needed 318 FTE primary care physicians integrated into the health system in our region.

These physicians have a long-term, full-time commitment to the University of Pennsylvania Health System (UPHS). They have clinical faculty appointments and meet a very high standard. This should allow us to cover about 1.4 million ambulatory visits or, if we were in a fully capitated system, about 600,000 covered lives.

We would need 237 FTE specialists and subspecialists to support that network, which would see approximately 710,000 specialty and subspecialty visits a year.

Our region spans up to Princeton in the northern part of Mercer County of New Jersey, to the Jersey Shore on the east, to the south down to Wilmington, Del., and to the west to Pottstown, Pa. We have identified the outstanding primary care physicians in this region to recruit into UPHS. We are currently in the process of negotiating with about 150 primary care physicians and have brought about 30 to closure as of this time. The program began last summer and is moving very rapidly.

We need this primary care network for our educational programs. We need a large number of primary care physicians to provide the ambulatory primary care experience for our students and residents that is the mandate of this era for education in medicine. We also need this network for our managed care programs.

This also will provide part of what we need for education in the various medical and surgical subspecialties as viewed by the relevant chairmen. We asked the chairman of each department, "What kind of patient flow do you need to have one of the top five academic programs in your discipline in graduate medical education?"

The numbers we got back from them are indicated in Table 2. The numbers that we would generate from our network visits as described above are indicated in the middle column.

When the difference, indicated in the last column, is positive, it shows that we have enough patients coming from just the network for this educational purpose. When the difference is negative, it means that we would have to have additional patients from other sources.

It is clear that we would need to continue to have access to patients outside of this network to meet the educational needs of a number of the surgical and medical subspecialties, for example, transplantation, neurosurgery, and oncology.

TABLE 2. *Comparison of projected network visits to educational (GME) need projections by Chairs*

Difference	Visits/1,000 in Calif. HMO	Network visits	FY 2000	Proj. needs
Primary care				
FP/internal medicine	1,613	956,805	Exceeds needs for GME	Exceeds needs for GME
Obstetrics/gynecology	345	204,763	Exceeds needs for GME	Exceeds needs for GME
Pediatrics	741	439,531	Exceeds needs for GME	Exceeds needs for GME
Specialties/subspecialties				
Dermatology	109	64,637	65,000	−373
Medicine	222	131,767	137,071	−5,254
Allergy/immunology	23	13,639	9,773	3,866
Cardiology	45	26,448	23,736	2,712
Endocrinology	16	9,726	27,528	−17,802
Gastroenterology	35	20,756	8,386	12,370
Hematology/oncology	37	22,060	29,929	−7,869
Infectious disease	12	7,353	4,887	2,466
Nephrology	29	16,960	14,240	2,720
Pulmonary medicine	25	14,825	10,914	3,911
Rheumatology	—	—	7,628	[−7,628]
Ophthalmology	169	99,920	85,000	14,920
Otorhinolaryngology	14	8,065	23,000	−14,935
Orthopedics	149	88,119	118,475	−30,356
Rehabilitation medicine	35	33,069	16,000	17,069
Psychiatry/psychology	55	32,615	80,000	−47,385
Surgery	261	154,773	60,352	47,036
Neurology	—	—	20,000	—

Note: Negative difference indicates additional patients needed; positive difference indicates excess of patients.

In addition, we believe this network will have an important impact on our research programs. For example, we believe we are in an era in which the explosion and understanding of the genetic basis of human disease will allow tremendous opportunities in the area of DNA diagnosis. It will also lead to the development of a whole new paradigm of how one counsels patients, shifting from prenatal diagnosis to adult counseling as we understand the genes related to breast cancer, colon cancer, and thousands of other diseases.

By systematic organization, we should be able to provide genetic counseling approaches and education, both for our patient population and our physicians, on how to implement the new genetics. This also provides an opportunity for intervention.

In addition, we have a strong health services research program, and this gives us a new patient population for that enterprise as well. We are looking at outcomes, new technologies, and different approaches.

As we enter the era of managed competition, I believe that some of the big events of the last 30 years in health care and its autonomy will pale by comparison to what we will experience over the next decade.

The implementation of clinical practice plans as part of an academic health center was necessary under Medicare. However, the cost was billions of dollars of lost revenue for those institutions that did not have practice plans and were slow in getting this done. It has also cost hundreds of millions of dollars in excess expenses for institutions that were unable to respond quickly to the implementation of DRGs in the mid-1980s.

If we cannot prepare for managed competition financially and try to stay ahead of the power curve, the results will be much more disastrous than they would have been in the past.

It is critical for us in academic health centers to recognize that academic excellence is our *raison d'etre*. That means we have to recruit and retain the best possible people and to provide the organization, the leadership, the support, and the financial resources to maximize the success of these people in pursuit of their mission within the AHC.

The Academic Health Center and Health
Care Reform, edited by R. Snyderman,
M.C. Rogers, and V.Y. Saito.
Raven Press, Ltd., New York © 1995.

Partner Attributes

James A. Lane, J.D.

The Kaiser Foundation Health Plan operates in 12 regions of the country, including North Carolina, and we have about 6.5 million members. We have over 9,000 physicians affiliated with our Permanente Medical Groups, 30 hospitals, and more than 220 medical office buildings.

Four of our regions are hospital-based; that is, they own and operate their own hospitals, but eight are not and they use one to three major hospitals in their areas. Most of the hospitals are teaching hospitals, e.g., the Cleveland Clinic.

Nine of our 12 regions use academic health centers in their regions for a variety of purposes. Those include Emory University, Kansas University, Georgetown University, UCSF, Stanford, and UCLA.

We also have a transplant program network that uses centers of excellence not only within our regions, but outside our regions, and, as I will discuss later, we base that on both cost and outcomes.

We have a teaching program that includes 600 residents in our major regions, and 3,000 M.D.s with clinical appointments at medical schools.

Interestingly enough, two of our regions were started by academic health centers. Our mid-Atlantic region, started by Georgetown University, had 50,000 members when we took over, and now it has more than 350,000 members. Kansas University started our Kansas City region, which we took over at 10,000 members and have now gotten up to 50,000 members.

We are seeking collaboration, partnership, and long-term relationships both in care delivery and in administrative support. We are particularly concerned about the patient management—the critical linkages as the patient leaves us and goes to the medical center and comes back.

We are interested in high quality services that can meet or beat our potential of real costs. In a number of cases we have stopped performing services because somebody else could provide them more efficiently than we could.

A third, and possibly the most important factor is good relationships with people. Our people and the people at the institution need to get along well, and often that is situational but can also become cultural.

Increasingly, we are looking for collaboration on quality-improvement projects. Most of our regions have embraced total quality management and are actively working on it. We look for those kinds of projects particularly in linkage areas where we and the health center interface.

Also, we are looking for innovative approaches, both for ourselves and for the health centers. One recent example is in Oregon, where our pediatric cardiologist does calls at Oregon University and he is covered by the OU physicians.

Finally, we are looking for low costs. A lot of people just look for discounts off of billed charges, but we consider the total package. There are multiple ways in which a relationship between ourselves and a medical center can result in low total costs, even though the unit costs are not as low as they might be otherwise. Those relate not only to the costs of the health care, but also to our physicians' costs and the time and effort that they have to spend in the relationship.

Our cultures do not always match, although we tend to have a more academic health center-like culture than a lot of other organizations. Our larger medical centers are organized and run like academic health centers, but we have different missions. We are a health care delivery system first. Education and research are secondary for us, which is not true for academic health centers.

Sometimes the health center is a state agency, adding to the complexity. Then we have two bureaucracies struggling with each other, which is often a problem. One conflict is over experimental procedures, a very touchy area for other insurance companies. We find health centers often pushing the envelope on their advice about whether a procedure is experimental.

I think it is important whether centers of excellence are perceived as voluntary or compulsory. There are efforts under way in health care reform to make them compulsory for health plans. As we look at centers of excellence in terms of both costs and outcomes, we shouldn't presume that academic health centers always have the best outcomes.

Here are two examples. The state of California has done a considerable amount of work on risk-adjusted outcomes and a long series on perinatal outcomes called the Williams Report. In that series, both Kaiser Permanente and other private nonprofit hospitals have better outcomes than the academic health centers in California. The same thing is true on risk-adjusted acute myocardial infarctions, where four of our hospitals (and no academic health centers) are among the top 10 in California.

In addition, we do not look at an academic health center as just a unit. We look at it service by service. Our hospitals that are very good on perinatal mortality are not necessarily the ones that are good on acute myocardial infarction, and this is true in academic health centers also. A series of studies shows that quality of care can vary at a given center from one service to another.

We use a variety of payment methods. We pay on a fee-for-service basis, sometimes discounted. We sometimes pay per diem, sometimes per case. I am not aware that we actually pay on a capitation basis, primarily because we are dealing mostly at the high end and it is very difficult to capitate those cases.

Capitation carries both the opportunity to gain and to lose. In any situation with capitation, when you take risks the down side always has to be considered.

In many of our regions we have very good relationships with academic health centers and are trying to strengthen those relationships. We clearly have need for very good outcomes on high-cost cases that we cannot provide ourselves and at low total costs.

There is the opportunity for us to provide other services, provided they are at the lowest cost, and this can be seen with our relationship with the Cleveland Clinic and an emerging relationship in Oregon. Once again, those have to be at the lowest total cost, and health centers have an advantage if you can package physician and hospital services together.

There is the question of owning your own HMO or setting up your own networks. We do participate with health centers that own their own HMOs. It is a minor part of their business. We are often a much bigger part of their business. You have to be careful and sensitive to discriminating in favor of your own HMO, because that will certainly discourage other plans.

We are also looking for opportunities for research and education relative to ambulatory health care delivery, to protocol development and dissemination, and to assessing the role of prevention and chronic care outcomes. Academic health centers have not necessarily focused on these areas, but a relationship with an organization like ours, which stresses primary health care delivery, can provide the opportunity to develop those fields.

Market forces are not only useful in creating efficiencies, but they also are important for allocating resources. The major policy debate appears to be about whether resources are going to be allocated primarily through central planning, which is a governmental function, or through market forces, or some combination of those two. It is important that we try to develop a system that can allocate resources through market mechanisms as much as possible.

The Academic Health Center and Health Care Reform, edited by R. Snyderman, M.C. Rogers, and V.Y. Saito. Raven Press, Ltd., New York © 1995.

Philosophies of Survival

Mitchell T. Rabkin, M.D.

It appears that some hospitals serve both as tertiary care referral centers and community hospitals, while others have much less of the community hospital function. Under health care reform, the former will probably tend to be more collegially involved in an integrated delivery network, whereas the latter will try to interact smoothly with one or more integrated delivery networks to secure specialty referrals only.

Those models represent two different philosophies of survival—the latter as hub and spoke, and the former a group of colleagues working together.

The goal of seamless progression of the individual patient will be met differently in those two organizational models. The more collegial arrangement will work to develop a common information system among all members. The latter may more likely sell discrete packages, such as cardiac catheterizations or bone marrow transplants, both to local integrated delivery systems and to national accounts, insurers, and employers.

Both of them may move residency rotations out to community hospitals and doctors' offices, and there will probably be a greater trend toward the apprenticeship role for training than we currently see, with more involvement of nurse practitioners and paraprofessionals.

Organization and business practices will change. When most of us trained in medicine, the concept of "hospital" could be visualized as a building with the outpatient area as a minor appendage. Now we think increasingly of a health system moving away from the episodic treatment of acute illness to dealing successfully over time with covered lives. Clearly, this change in function requires a parallel change in organization.

We face a struggle, because we have been brought up in a world of fee-for-service and cost reimbursement in which we were promised and usually found a rose garden, and now we confront real-world conditions where there is no guarantee at all.

Health care reform could make things better or worse, but the pressure of today's buyer's market—well before any health care reform emerges from Capitol Hill—mandates management thinking that is unprecedented for academic health centers. It is not simply a question of cutting personnel or revising systems. Our goals relate to service and scholarship. We hope to stay solvent, as opposed to investor-owned organizations in business to make money by delivering health care. Our challenge relates not only to becoming more business-like, but how to do so with preservation of those missions of scholarship, quality, innovation, and care of the uninsured as well.

One major problem is that the ratcheting down of prices by government decreases the margins we are used to paying. It means fewer resources for cost shifting are available to the hospital director and to the dean.

One major change in organization many of us are struggling with has to do with information systems management. Some hospitals have reasonably successful systems for clinical information management, and some have begun to integrate these with financial management.

Most information systems leave a great deal to be desired with respect to today's management needs. Tomorrow we will need to know the cost and clinical behavior of individual physicians and the characteristics of the way institutions deal with each clinical situation so we can negotiate.

We want to incorporate ways to document quality. We want to use the computer to help educate and foster behavior that contributes to improved quality. Then, subsequently, we need to create an information system that oversees many institutions in an integrated delivery network and to look at these same events collectively in terms of how the entire network is serving its clients.

Finally, this needs to be done so that it is easier rather than more difficult for doctors to practice medicine and so that the intellectual and personal gratifications of the profession are restored. That is what attracts the best people to medicine.

An information management system that can accomplish all this in ways that inform and support our strategic planning requires sophisticated technology. It also calls for an executive leader in information systems management, which is relatively novel for the academic medical center and perhaps for most organizations as well.

We have discussed external forces in the environment creating business pressures, needs for networking, and information requirements. Internal forces for change exist within the hospital as well. Today's academic chairman faces a tougher time getting research grants, problems related to increasing diversity and geographic spread of the milieu for teaching, and the resulting problems that include controlling quality and monitoring curriculum.

By virtue of the nature of the health care business today, this academician increasingly must be a part of top administration, whereas years ago he or she did not need to be. He or she simply needed to be satisfied with the way the administration ran the hospital.

The demands on time for chiefs-of-service are intensifying rapidly. Each chairman will have to organize his or her respective departments to meet these demands, and this is particularly difficult for the larger departments like medicine and surgery.

In addition to that, there is the question of excellence, which, in the past, was defined along one vector—professional excellence. And, who defined it? Each individual academician, each individual doctor did. "If they all practice medicine the way I practice, there would be no health care problem!" This antediluvian attitude prevailed until recently, but it is fast eroding.

Go beyond that single vector and create a two-dimensional graph. One dimension is technical excellence, and the other is systems efficiency. You can be a great surgeon, but if you schedule your patient for 8 AM, and you show up at 8:30 AM, and you throw the expensive instruments on the floor, and you take 3.5 hours when you've booked 2, you're ruining the system for yourself and for everybody else.

That dimension is characterized by a marvelous cartoon. The patient says, "Doctor, I just feel so badly about bothering you." And the doctor says, "Madam, you don't understand. You are revenue, and I am expense."

A third dimension called personal expectations should be considered for all-round performance. As length of stay shortens, conditions become more hectic, and patients are pushed around by the consequences of economic pressures in health care, we are learning that patients' personal expectations have to be met. Doctors' personal expectations have to be met as well. Employees' expectations are also important. This is a dramatic change in the way academic health centers have operated, and the struggle is just beginning.

How do you create the kinds of organizations that really influence, monitor, and control the way things operate? That is one of the internal challenges we have for the future.

What are the practical politics of all of this? Lobbyists from diverse groups are traveling to Washington trying to exert an influence. There is a relative diffidence of academic faculty to write and to call and to visit, and yet, those letters and those visits do make a difference. In meetings on Capitol Hill, I have heard repeatedly, "Well, I haven't heard very much about it. I don't think the academicians care about this."

Most congressmen do not hear enough from all of us in academic medicine, while everyone else is at the table pounding with their spoons. We have to recognize we are not only entering the real world of economics, but the real world of politics as well.

The Academic Health Center and Health Care Reform, edited by R. Snyderman, M.C. Rogers, and V.Y. Saito. Raven Press, Ltd., New York © 1995.

Swimming in the Same Sea

David W. Singley, Jr.

My message is that no matter what each of us does, we all swim in the same sea. This means I am probably going to encounter you, and we are going to work together or compete.

Coastal Physician Services Group, Inc. is a publicly-traded national physicians' group providing diversified practice management services to physicians and physician groups. The main purpose of our services is to help physicians move from being providers of care to managers of care.

At Coastal, our revenue in 1993 was in the neighborhood of $450 million, and next year it will be in excess of $700 million. The environment we see is that of the $940 billion spent on health care; with the movement to outpatient services, approximately $175-$200 billion will be spent on physician services.

Roughly one-half of that can be consolidated into large physician groups. Groups such as Coastal, Phycor, and Pacific Physician Services represent approximately only $1 billion in that market. There is a tremendous opportunity to consolidate what we consider a cottage industry into a major force in the future of health care.

When Coastal was founded, it provided hospital-based physician services such as emergency medicine, anesthesiology, and obstetrics. Coastal has recently expanded rapidly into acquiring primary care practices and primary care networks, with the ability to take full risk for a given patient population. In this model, the physician group is responsible for the entire well-being of a group of Medicare and commercial HMO enrollees. This includes delivering all primary care services, all specialty, subspecialty, hospital, and all ancillary care.

The key here is that an HMO has ceded the risk to us, and, as a physicians' group, we are going to provide the primary care services ourselves and then decide whom we are going to use in terms of quality and costs for all the other health care needs.

This is sometimes called a physician-equity model, and it is clearly an opportunity for a physician group to stand shoulder-to-shoulder with both insurance companies and hospitals in playing an integrator role in the future of health care.

The organization and business practice of health care delivery are rapidly changing and, quite frankly, gravitating toward the most efficient models of care.

From many of the for-profit health care conferences held on Wall Street and throughout the country, you learn a tremendous amount. We saw one model involving a hip replacement done at an outpatient surgery center where the patient never entered the hospital. Following surgery, the patient is moved to a nursing home with a critical care unit, and then to another side of the nursing home.

With this type of model, the per diem cost of hospital stay would be cut in half—from the neighborhood of $700 to $350 a day. The impact of that added revenue is powerful.

Quality is an issue for a physician group. Our group is set up to allow practitioners to govern the quality and clinical care.

There is a clear place in business for this type of health care, and, if a company can raise capital on Wall Street and return earnings, it will be a force and will compete with everyone else out in the sea.

The future of our health care delivery is about picking partners or otherwise risk being excluded. The idea that academic health care centers are impervious to market forces due to their special position of research, training, and tertiary care is no longer valid. There may not be any patients coming to academic health centers if someone buys up all the primary care centers in town.

Well-capitalized groups such as Coastal have the ability to consolidate the cottage industry of physician practices and thus control large patient populations that academic health care centers may have previously depended upon.

Physicians are looking to the future with fear, anxiety, and trepidation and, thus, looking to form associations. Their choices are hospitals, insurance companies and, finally, physician groups.

Dr. Rogers' previous comments about how insurance companies can get into the physician side of the business easier than physicians can get into the insurance side of the business is up for debate. Working with physicians is not as easy as it seems. In over 15 years of working with doctors in very difficult circumstances, we have found the ability to recruit, retain, and attract high quality physicians is paramount.

If I create a model that is attractive, I do not necessarily have to buy all the practices. I can recruit physicians from academic health care centers or anywhere else. I have to have the ability either to buy or build.

So the question really becomes, Can the academic health care center join the three categories that I claim will be integrators in the future—hospitals, insurance companies and physician groups? Can an academic health center become an integrator, create an integrated health care delivery system in any given geographic market? I think the answer is, Perhaps.

Certainly, the new parameters of cost and efficiency must be balanced with the primary missions that have been service, tertiary care, training, and research. Funding for academic health care centers that do not integrate is a tough road. It will be political, because the choices are essentially legislative—standing up before God and country and saying, "We deserve a legislative carve-out. We deserve funding just because of who we are, regardless of market forces."

It will require fund-raising that will incorporate being a competitive health plan. Instead of cost-shifting, it will require profit-shifting from the profit side of the business of delivering quality care in a cost-effective manner to the missions of research and training.

Our company appears to threaten a lot of people. When we bought the primary care practices in South Florida, we accounted for 65% of the admissions in one of the Columbia hospitals, and, almost immediately, we got a great deal of attention and respect.

That is what is happening with insurance companies and with hospitals. I believe that a physician-equity model that stands up shoulder-to-shoulder to the other elements of the delivery system will be part of the future.

The Academic Health Center and Health Care Reform, edited by R. Snyderman, M.C. Rogers, and V.Y. Saito. Raven Press, Ltd., New York © 1995.

Responses

Joseph B. Martin, M.D., Ph.D.: From the perspective of an academic health center, the situation in Northern California is in a state of flux. In the past 3 or 4 years, we have had essentially 50% of our patients under managed care. This includes more than 120 contracts put together primarily by the medical center, the medical school, and the medical practice group, comprising about 900 physicians.

That group has been in place for 8 years, but it has become clear within the past year that the tertiary care referrals are falling off. This is not because our physicians are not as good as they used to be or that physicians do not want to refer their patients but because there are many constraints of the referral patterns.

In the past 6 months, we have formed the Clinical Strategies Committee, co-chaired by the dean of the medical school and the director of the hospital, to consider what the future will bring.

We have merged with one community hospital and are focusing intently on networking to assure tertiary care referrals. At the same time, we are building a primary care base and thinking about how we can capitate both Medicare and, in California, Medicaid. The Medicaid population will become capitated over the next couple of years.

We are interested in two major regions. One is the San Francisco area, where we would have our relationship to the county hospital, San Francisco General Hospital. The other area is the Central San Joaquin Valley, where our Fresno program, which is an outlier program in primary care, will also be actively involved in the managed care or capitated care of the Medicaid population.

The structural changes we are considering can be most dramatically represented by our emerging approach to both cancer and to cardiology.

Our cardiology group, which includes the internal medicine cardiologists, the cardiac surgeons, and the interventional neuroradiologists or cardiac radiologists, wants to work both in the inpatient and in the outpatient area as a group.

With departmental boundaries broken down, the principal problem that we have in tertiary care referral, in an area such as this or in cancer, is that of the patient not finding entry to our system user-friendly. They require multiple visits. They come to see the cardiologist. They get referred to the x-ray department a week later. They then come back to see the cardiac surgeon a week later. We are very eager to put in place a one-visit-see-everybody-you-need-to-see plan.

We have formed a breast cancer clinic where the clinician interested in breast cancer, together with the surgeon and the oncologist, can see the patient the same day, determine what the best treatment will be, and by the end of the day the patient knows what the next step will be.

These events have caused us to consider, for example, the role of a chairman of a department of medicine in the new world. The traditional role of the academic leader, who is an expert researcher, a wonderful teacher, and a fine clinician, probably will not survive in the future.

The individual who will deliver the kind of quality care in a competitive market in a consumer-friendly way is a different role model than the individual who is successful in getting NIH grants and at the traditional academic roles that we have revered for so long. As we move to search for a new chair of our department of medicine, we may consider an alternative role model.

There is movement toward relating our academic activities in internal medicine closely to our strong interdepartmental programs in basic science and to make the clinical activities be competitive in the marketplace.

The residency reductions mandated in the State of California have caused considerable rethinking among our subspecialty departments about how we will deliver service with fewer residents. In neurosurgery, an effective plan is already in place that allows nurse practitioners to deliver much of the standard care that residents used to deliver more efficiently. We will be training more nurse practitioners to work with us in the academic settings.

The change is so rapid that its impact on us is almost stunning. Although anxiety is high, excitement is high as well. There is a great deal of interest in innovative approaches.

Gary A. Mecklenburg, M.B.A.: As either hospitals or academic health centers, we are working in a competitive marketplace that is moving fast and is dominated by market forces.

If we expect to receive the revenue associated with a service organization, then we are going to have to play by the rules of the competitive marketplace whether we like them or not. Academic centers have to make a case to our friends in Washington to try and have those elements of our mission protected and funded. However, on the service side, we are going to have to do the same things that everybody does.

From my point of view as a hospital administrator in Chicago, I see certain assumptions and factors critical for success. First, we are going to be in a managed-care marketplace moving toward being responsible for the health of a defined population at a predetermined, fixed price.

Capitation is going to look awfully good to us pretty soon, because the ratcheting down on discounted per diems and fee-for-service will intensify. Academic centers will not get much extra capitation compared to everybody else. That also mandates being part of a regional delivery system.

At Northwestern Health Care Network, our goal is to be responsible for 1.5

million covered lives in metropolitan Chicago by the year 2000. To do that requires a system of hospitals, but fewer hospitals. We are really talking about providers—physicians and alternative delivery sites.

I agree with Jim Mulvihill's critical success factors of price–price–price–service–quality. We are in a price-driven marketplace.

Chicago is different than Durham. Both cities are different than New York, which is different than San Diego. The health care reform will evolve slightly differently in each area, but some of the principles are the same.

To be successful, we believe we have to have an integrated clinical enter-prise—hospitals and physicians coming together economically, where success and failure are inextricably linked. The separateness of physicians and hospitals in health care cannot continue.

We believe that in our system we have to have about 900 primary care phy-sicians who are full-time equivalents. A full-time equivalent is a primary care physician who has to be efficient at taking responsibility for between 2,000 and 2,500 covered lives.

Geographic coverage is essential. If you are going to cover 1.5 million covered lives as we are, you have to have health care where people are. That includes the doctors, emergency departments, and obstetrical services.

Cost management and utilization management are paramount, and that ap-pears to be our Achilles' heel. I do not think we are going to be able to defend our higher cost structure over the long term. A lot of work is being done in that regard, but we have to move a lot faster.

In response to the question about insurance, we gave up a long time ago on the thought of setting up our own managed care product. If you were an early entrant, it would be possible, but as far as I can tell the industry has consoli-dated. I do not want to compete head-to-head with people that have billions of dollars in cash to try and set up our own insurance coverage. So, our strategy is to cooperate.

A critical success factor is that you have to have a governance and manage-ment structure that can make it work. My experience at four different academic medical centers suggests that most of them cannot move fast and cannot make quick decisions. This needs to be addressed.

The unwieldy committee structure of academic health centers and the 1 to 1.5-year search process to recruit a clinical leader cannot continue.

At the Northwestern Health Care Network, we have worked for the last 6 years to put together a regional delivery system. As of November, it became permanent after a 3-year trial period. We integrated Northwestern Memorial, Children's Memorial, Evanston, and Highland Park Hospitals under a com-mon holding company. We anticipate seven to ten hospitals within the next 18 months or so.

A critical success factor for the future is access to capital. We are replacing facilities right now. We are about to break ground on a project that will cost about $700 million.

In the health care reform movement, there is a failure to recognize the need for capital and the capital replacement cycle. For those of you who have newer facilities, consider that in a decade you will need new ones.

The investment in new technology is another consideration. Where are you going to get the capital to purchase new technology if you do not generate profits? Fund-raising is important but cannot cover all the costs.

Just as the Wall Street marketplace looks at for-profit companies like Coastal, they are also assessing you, and, if you cannot match up with the marketplace, you will not get loan money on Wall Street.

Capital is an entirely different matter for our long-term future. Whether you are investing in practices, new buildings, or new technology, you need capital, and we have a potential problem of being starved for capital in the next decade or so.

Bruce J. Sams, M.D.: As a friend of academic health centers and a member of the clinical faculty at UCSF for 30 years, I have noted with great interest and some concern that programs like Kaiser Permanente have inadvertently provided a problem for academia. As you well know, the domination of a service area by managed care presents AHCs with the most serious challenge they have faced in several decades. Competition will be good, but not easy, for American medicine. I have great faith that the leadership in AHCs will find the right path for their institutions and that they will be stronger and more pertinent teachers of medicine because of the broadened responsibility for patient care which will ensue.

I would like to comment on some specific aspects of the changes facing you, based on my experience in managed care. First of all, the ambulatory sector will replace the hospital as the center of the AHC universe. This shift in focus is extremely hard for many to accept, yet it is essential to survival. Mankind has come to accept that the earth is not the center of our larger universe—perhaps we can also accept the same view of the hospital. Systems designed primarily to support the hospital, at the expense of the ambulatory sector, will be too expensive to survive. If we care for patients outside of the hospital, then much of our teaching, as well as research, must follow.

Another crucial change for AHCs will be finding patient members for your system that are as healthy as the average member of the community, or failing that, finding a way to identify and be compensated for sicker patients. Obviously, large centers providing excellent care for cancer, heart disease, and other serious conditions will most likely attract patients who need or anticipate a need for this care. On the other hand, community-based plans will attract the young who want easy access to episodic routine care.

As managed care dominates a community, you may well find that community physicians are less available for teaching. As physicians see their incomes leveling off or falling, and the AHCs competing with them for patients, they well may lose interest. In Kaiser Permanente, we have had to depend primarily on interested physicians donating their time for teaching. It is hard to build teaching time into doctors' schedules and still be competitive with plans that do not. Buyers of health care have not been willing to pay more for health insurance simply to subsidize teaching programs; consequently, teaching costs are rarely identified and discussed explicitly with buyers.

I recognize the strong temptation to develop managed care programs that cause a minimum of distress among the faculty. Unfortunately, such plans often do not involve enough change to be effective, and the resulting failure of the plan can be terminal. Self-deception is as dangerous here as in other areas of life.

Capitated, vertically integrated systems are maximally cost-effective when the elements of the system (hospital beds, generalists, specialists, offices) are in balance. AHCs usually do not start off in this balanced state. You should make the best possible estimates of the size of the patient population you will serve, and derive your estimated needs from these figures. For instance, if you already have more beds than needed, bringing more hospitals into the "network" simply worsens your bed surplus. These same hospitals that may send some tertiary care cases will be your competitors for secondary care. Admittedly, win-win arrangements can be found, but all of the ramifications of these networks must be understood before getting into the deal.

Physician behavior is probably the major determinant of success or failure in capitated plans. Physicians control 80% of the budget. Patient satisfaction, quality, and access are heavily dependent on physician activity.

Kaiser Permanente has recognized the central role of physicians for 50 years and continues to place a very high value on physician participation in the management of the program. If a managed care system must rely on micromanagement of physicians by nonphysicians, it is unlikely to survive over the long run. The greatest attention must be given to structuring the system correctly in the first place, so that physicians will want it to succeed and will behave accordingly.

The Academic Health Center and Health Care Reform, edited by R. Snyderman, M.C. Rogers, and V.Y. Saito. Raven Press, Ltd., New York © 1995.

General Discussion

Moderator Rogers: When we talk about excellence, we are not referring to buildings. We are talking about faculty members. Ninety-nine percent of our faculty practice is in their facility, and the internal composition and size of the facility is going to change.

How do we define excellence with regard to faculty presently? How do we define excellence with regard to faculty in the future? How do we get there?

Dr. Relman: I would like to hear some discussion about the comment that academic health centers simply could not and, even implied, should not get into competition with the big insurance companies or the new physician–management companies in the establishment of HMOs or managed care products of one kind or another.

The approach that seems to be taken by Bill Kelley at the University of Pennsylvania and Gary Mecklenburg at Northwestern is, yes, we can compete with insurers in some way.

Gary appears to believe that we have to make a deal with the insurance companies. Does that mean that you will let the insurance companies market and deliver your patients, take a piece off the top, and you provide the comprehensive services with your staff and facilities and share some of the risk?

Mr. Mecklenburg: There are various components of the future health care delivery system, two of which are the provider component and the insurance component.

You can basically form your own insurance company. Should we do that? There was an opportunity to enter the HMO or PPO business 10 years ago in most marketplaces when the market was fragmented and the cost of entry was not high. Today, as I look around the country, the market is consolidated, the cost of entry is huge, and I do not believe that most of us have either the expertise or the capital to compete in that business.

They have to want to work with you. It involves the price–price– price–price–service–quality issue because they are the ones who will sell your services. They will also take something off the top and try to regulate your behavior. The alternative is not to have access to the patients we serve and the revenue that comes with that.

Dr. Relman: Who takes the risk?

Mr. Mecklenburg: That is another fascinating issue. Much of what is going on in health care reform is transferring risk. Where the risk is shifting, folks, is right to us. We will commit to providing the care on some kind of capitated basis and, therefore, we will be taking the risk.

Dr. Kelley: In the future, the money is going to be in the HMO. U.S. Health Care, for example, spent $.72 on every $1 for physicians, hospitals, and administration, and the other $.28 is used at their discretion. To me, that is an important variable to be considered.

I do not know whether we should go the route of an independent HMO or a joint venture, but we are going to have to do something. We are dealing with very aggressive, effective, competent, large organizations with a great deal of money and clout. They can put tremendous pressure on us, particularly in our market where there are only two dominant HMOs. It is very hard to negotiate with both of them.

Dr. Pardes: The common wisdom is that the bulk of academic health centers cannot be on that management side, simply for the reasons articulated by Gary Mecklenburg and Bill Kelley. You need an amount of capital that most academic health centers do not have and also you will be competing head-to-head with companies. If you compete with these other companies, they have every reason not to want to do business with you for other health care possibilities. Basically, you restrict yourself to one company.

Is it a fair statement that the overwhelming number of academic health centers will not consider the option, will set themselves up with the ability to provide a network that is purchasable, and then will go to companies to either co-venture or to have their services purchased?

Dr. Schroeder: Just a point of clarification. Two-thirds of the academic medical centers in this country are state schools, which may have actual restrictions from being able to raise this kind of capital and enter into those kind of arrangements.

Dr. Langfitt: It seems to me that the very distinguished academic health centers that have spawned reputations and tremendous connections within their particular region ought to associate with very large distinguished rich insurance companies.

The large insurance companies are insuring millions of lives, and in their group insurance programs they have millions of people who are in indemnity insurance. Now, they recognize that the system is going to shift to capitation also, and they are wondering what they will do about all these indemnity plans that they have.

Rather than the academic health center going its independent way, it seems prudent to establish some partnerships up front in the beginning.

This is not going to be easy, obviously, because the insurance company and the academic health center are coming from opposite ends of the spectrum and are not going to understand each other very well.

In the process of putting a partnership together and acquiring primary care practices, simultaneously, the insurance company would be trying to position itself. It might begin by buying some local HMOs, establishing its own HMO, or using its indemnity position within a particular region to try to convert them to a capitated program. This would form, in effect, a core of the patient service system for the academic health center.

The doctors could continue to do fee-for-service around the edges of this capitated system for as long as the fee-for-service system seemed to pay off, but they would be working in concert with this partner. Over time, you could gradually expand that covered patient base with the partner putting in much of the required capital. This core service system, the accountable health plan, will gradually expand, possibly over a decade or two, and account for virtually the entire service system for the academic health center in a partnership with this large insurance company.

Dr. Martin: Although we have not explicitly said it, most of us who exist in large urban centers are competing with each other. Our academic health centers are not only struggling in the managed care business, but we are undercutting each other at the same time in the pricing of the services we currently depend on the most.

Until we come to grips with the fact that most of our major centers have too many hospital beds and that too many hospitals are struggling, the networks that you are discussing will have some trouble bringing themselves into focus.

In San Francisco, our occupancy rates in hospitals now are well below 50%, and the hospitals are refusing to shut down. Some of them will have to close before one can really get such a system to work.

Dr. Robinson: There is tremendous first-entry advantage to the institution that wishes to take a capitated product to market in an immature market. The cost goes up as that market matures.

In our own market, which is relatively immature, we do have a capitated plan that we are taking to the small businesses in a relatively rural state. It is designed for them, with an infrastructure that is now being sought to service other groups in our region.

There is no way that we can build sufficient covered lives through operation of our own capitated plan within a reasonable time frame to achieve all of our goals. Taking equity positions, so that we are at the table with other plans and products in our region, is another part of our strategy and is beginning to work well. We are now buying into a 225,000 covered-lives product in our region that would make us an equal partner in terms of policies.

I predict that as our markets mature, we will see coalescence of these products over time. At present, we are more or less competing with ourselves.

In other product lines, we are only a player, and one of our objectives is to try to maintain sufficient market share and sufficient dominance in our market-place so that people will want to do business with us as they come into our region.

In the future, as increased amounts of risk are transferred to our institutions by the marketplace, our parent universities may wish to isolate their patient care arms from the rest of the university to protect the College of Arts & Science from that risk.

This situation is beginning to require us to choose a partner, to choose alliances, and to eliminate others. We can no longer serve everybody, and I find that very unsettling. I do not believe that exclusivity is a function of the university. It is one of the unfortunate prices that seem to be exacted from a traditional university system, and it is difficult to change the culture.

Looking at our in-hospital environment, our faculty have embraced reduction of utilization with such force that we are reducing revenues so rapidly that we can hardly keep up on the expense side.

Dr. Kelley: In Philadelphia, we have a microcosm of the country. One recent example is that Independence Blue Cross of Eastern Pennsylvania has basically acquired the Graduate Health System and is clearly becoming its own provider organization. Graduate Health System encompasses 1,200 plus beds and seven hospitals, basically a hospital that spun off from the University of Pennsylvania about 15 years ago and has had its own HMO for some 15 years. It used to be our HMO when it was set up in the middle 1970s, but it moved with Graduate Hospital when they separated from us. If Independence Blue Cross is successful in becoming a payor-provider organization, we are likely to see many other health insurance organizations doing basically the same thing.

With regard to managed care, if one is strong enough to achieve a true joint venture relationship with a health insurance organization, then that may be the best approach in many markets. However, if one is not strong enough to deal as an equal partner, one will be acquired, and that would not be acceptable to our trustees or to most of us.

Dr. Mulvihill: There probably will be 126 different solutions to meet the specific needs of each of our academic health centers. But a critical mass of population is necessary to be one of the top two or three players in that region. The academic center will probably have to be one of the two or three lowest-cost providers in a region. If the center is not the lowest, the cost should be made up by quality.

We have talked a lot about partnerships between AHCs and insurance companies and managed care entities. It may be that more than two entities will enter a joint venture or an alliance. It may be two academic health centers in a city. It may be some of the companies dealing with information, whether they are the consulting firms or the Baby Bells and the communications companies.

Dr. Waller: It appears that the alternative to enter the competition is to risk downsizing to the point that we lose critical mass to fulfill our important missions—education and research. I am encouraged that academic health centers can, in fact, compete.

Dr. Petersdorf: For state universities to be able to compete, particularly those that own university hospitals, they will have to divest themselves of their hospitals or find other ways to separate the hospital from the university.

I want to reiterate that if physician groups are to succeed, particularly faculty physician groups, they will have to become more involved and knowledgeable about management.

   The numbers provided by Bill Kelley demonstrate a clear shortage of primary care physicians, but there must be too many specialists. If only a limited number of specialists is needed, what will happen to all the excess specialists?

   I also do not understand how the program will be funded. Perhaps Bill can enlighten us as to where the capital is coming from to drive the admirable program that you have instituted.

   Dr. Kelley: We believe that 237 FTE subspecialists will be required to service the primary care network. The FTEs are practicing full-time, and virtually none of our academic specialists and subspecialists practice full-time. They all teach or conduct research. We have about 275 clinical FTEs right now from our 610 faculty, which is the number of full-time faculty in the practice plans. That is a separate number from the numbers necessary for us to continue to be one of the top five academic training programs in each of the specialties.

   We need to have additional carve-outs from other sources, other HMOs, or other programs. We cannot support the kind of subspecialty training programs we want to have in neurosurgery, transplantation, and oncology through a primary care network with 600,000 capitated lives.

   Currently, we are able to support the capital requirements almost entirely through the hospital resource. We have committed $100 million to developing the network. We can support that now through the hospital, but we probably will not be able to 5 years from now. We are trying to get the program established while we have some capital.

   A critical element is that the school and the hospital are together in one organization, so that we can use those funds to do what is best for the institution without a lot of debate about who benefits and who does not.

   Dr. Relman: I hope we do not forget the essential fact that everything we are discussing depends on physicians. We are best able to appeal to physicians. We talk to them about the profession they believe in and why they chose medicine. Capital may be important, but even more important than capital are the physicians, and they bring the patients. Start from our own physicians and those in the community, whom we have educated and inspired and whom we can attract to practice in relation to the academic health center.

   There is no question that the changing organization of health care requires physicians to practice in groups and on the capitated basis. We have to have multispecialty groups, and we have to be dependent on a very large cadre of primary care physicians. The question is: Who is going to own and manage those physicians?

   What worries me about physician-management organizations or insurance company-owned organizations is that the fundamental professional responsibility of physicians to decide what should be done with their patients is in jeopardy.

   I know that the business organizations that are recruiting physicians are saying, "We are not going to practice medicine. We will let you practice medicine the way you want."

However, they tell their investors that they will keep medical loss ratios down to make it attractive. That will enable them to aggrandize the organization and have all the executives and corporate activities that are valued so highly.

In order to do that, they have to control what the physicians do. If physicians are managed by businesses with the best of intentions and with the best of the claims, medicine will be deprofessionalized, and physicians will sell their souls to the market. That is not why we entered the medical profession.

The question is, Can capital be gotten and costs controlled as well as the insurance company can but with not-for-profit professional management? I am firmly convinced that this can be done, because there are examples of it being done now.

If we do not draw a line in the sand now, once that medical/industrial complex is in place and big money is being made, it will be a long time before the American health care system finds its soul again.

Is price really what we are worried about, or is it total cost? I am not aware of any industrial market where the total amount of money spent by the consumer on the product is of concern to the manufacturers or to the vendors. They want to expand their market by having an attractive price but not to reduce the total amount of money spent by society on their product. The goal is to increase the total amount of money spent on their product by segmenting the market, selling more, advertising, and inventing new, fancy gimmicks and boutiques.

If we buy into the myth that by making us more price-sensitive, the marketplace will reduce the amount of money that America spends on health care, this is tantamount to believing in the "tooth fairy." You have to believe that these various corporations will get to a certain point and say, "Look, our total revenues have reached $2 billion. We don't want any more because if we increase our revenues beyond $2 billion, America will be spending too much on health care." That is not going to happen.

Dr. Schroeder: Academic medicine faces a collective management challenge, and I would ask: Can it hold together?

Several discussants have pointed out the need for a united front in Washington to try to get a big piece of the pie. However, there are tremendous fragmentary forces at work.

One is that there are great differences in the capacity to raise capital among the 126 academic centers. Secondly, within most of our major urban centers, there is intensifying competition taking place in a substrate with excess capacity of hospital beds and specialty capability. That excess will have to shrink. It is hard to have solidarity when you want to put the other fellow out of business.

There is disagreement about the desired educational product, and there is the public/private issue. I wonder whether the center can hold, or whether the better-off academic medical centers will split off (like HIAA) because they feel they can better represent themselves. If that happens it will hamper the ability to speak with one voice. I believe we need to pay attention to this, because there is probably already some splintering.

There is a tendency to think of partnership as a one-time solution—"Boy, if we could only find a partner, or enter some kind of relationship, we would be home free!" The business pages show that there are acquisitions and divestments, and contracts last for a year or two. You can be taken over by a company that then gets taken over by another company, who looks at this product and says, "I don't want you to be in this—out!"

Dr. Snyderman: The focus here seems to be a whole new concept of how health care will be delivered. A lot of this is based on the new economics of health care reimbursement. These trends lead to moving away from taking care of sick people and moving toward taking care of the health of large populations.

The academic health center has always been focused on taking care of sick people. If we are dealing with sick people, then clearly, we are the center of health care delivery.

If you start thinking of taking care of large populations and their health, you then need to visualize a very different system with networks and all the elements we have discussed. The academic health center plays a very different role.

To take care of the health of a large population, geographic location will dictate our role to some degree. Durham, North Carolina, has a different population density than Nashville, Philadelphia, San Francisco, or New York. It may very well be that we could develop meaningful or appropriate partners of 500,000 lives. The University of Pennsylvania may be able to serve 1.5 million.

We have characteristically judged excellence of the top five or ten academic health centers not only by their excellence but also by the scope of their operation. The new scales will drive us to do things that will distort the models we need to consider. It may be very difficult, depending on your population base, to support an entity as big as it takes to be one of the top five or top ten medical centers in the United States. Academic centers should begin thinking about redefining excellence sooner rather than later.

Professor Reinhardt: Ten years ago when we met here, there was great alarm over the future of the academic health center under the pro-competitor strategy in the Reagan era, where it was thought that your patients would be sensitive to price. A lot of us really did not believe there was a problem. In fact, it was a negative problem. The academic health center quickly discovered that the private payers were patsies, and they would pay for anything.

In the process, the academic medical centers really did discover a "cash cow" and milked it thoroughly. Now, as I understand it, there is this academic health center business, and there is excess capacity in that business. In America, or anywhere in the world, there are only two approaches to reduce excess.

One is through coordination, called planning with government, with the government orchestrating the table manners. The alternative, which is the American way, is that you turn this over to some hard-nosed private entrepreneurs who know how to push people around and who are paid enormously well for this dirty work. Somehow entrepreneurs are respected and government people are not.

I believe it is not like 10 years ago, when some of us said, "They're crying wolf." This time you really are at the crossroads. One model could be that you are a national resource and should be nationally supported, but at a level that is considered appropriate in the political process, and then every one of these competing health plans has access to you. You are not aligned with one of them, but you serve all of them because you are the frontier of medicine. Then you can function like the old traditional academic health center, but downsized.

The alternative is that you turn it over to private entrepreneurs. The reason they get rich is because they know how to reduce excess capacity. That is basically what all of them are doing, squeezing out the fat, and taking a good chunk in their own pocket.

There may be, in fact, a parting of the ways; some centers might prefer one road and others prefer another road. You can curse private entrepreneurs, but if we do not like the government, it is the only recourse available.

Dr. Weldon: We are hearing a potential clash of two cultures. Business has learned painfully to constantly come to grips with change. The painful removal of "fat" that business is going through is not the end.

We have to learn from some of the new experiments to become a better instrument to manage more effective and rapid change while maintaining the best of the old culture. We also need to look at the opportunities for diversity.

Moderator Rogers: In the 1980s, when the telephone industry broke up Ma Bell, no one understood completely that we would have the telephone, the television, the satellite, the computer, and other means of communication as part of one system, which includes Time Warner and other communications businesses.

The ability to see over the horizon was beyond the level of expertise of their best people. It should not embarrass us or frighten us to understand that the kind of fundamental change ongoing in the health care industry will result in complex realignments that are beyond our ability to comprehend fully. There cannot be one simple answer to this. It will evolve into models that we cannot yet even contemplate.

The Academic Health Center and Health
Care Reform, edited by R. Snyderman,
M.C. Rogers, and V.Y. Saito.
Raven Press, Ltd., New York © 1995.

Session IV: Conference Summary and Reflections

Dealing With the Inefficiencies

William G. Anlyan, M.D.

The world is changing, and the academic health center has to change with it. I support the plans of going from the self-contained academic health center to a Duke Health System and the analogs at other institutions. Flexibility and ability to change have been the hallmarks of the leading academic health centers in this country.

There are multiple options: Be independent, be part of a merger or a joint venture, as well as other approaches. The choice will depend on the individual academic health center.

We have to trim the inefficiencies of research and education. For example, you cannot compete with a Mayo Clinic when you have three physical exams and history takings by the student, the resident, and the attending physician.

A major problem that has not been addressed here is the fit with your university, not just the hospital and the medical school. There has traditionally been a classical problem of fitting the inefficiencies of the university. There has always been that back door of "establishing a level playing field," where monies have gone from the academic health center to the university. I believe that bears re-examination.

I propose having the universities become more like corporations; that is a much bigger, tougher change than what we are looking at today. I do not know if American Airlines or any other airline could form a profit by operating for 6 or 7 months of the year on 3 or 4 days a week. We have a bigger job with our mother universities in terms of efficiency and not being an additional financial drain as we enter the competitive world.

Tenure is another problem. It is not going to be possible for one institution to get rid of tenure. I would hope that a cluster of academic health centers, the leading ones, would examine this because tenure is a source of dead wood as you try to get rid of the excess in the academic health center.

There is no question that downsizing the faculty is another important consideration. Just last week, I talked at the American Surgical Association meeting about assessing the Ph.D. production in the basic sciences. The average basic science faculty member produces 15 Ph.D. candidates, each one of whom thinks they should be competing successfully for NIH grants.

99

Clearly, decision-making needs be expedited. In my own time, I have believed that an oligarchy was the best form of governance of the academic medical center, while we pretend it to be as democratic as possible.

The topic of ownership of the teaching hospital has been raised, and I have a biased point of view. It has been a tremendous, wonderful asset at Duke University to be able to have the teaching hospital included in the same corporation.

I have served for 10 years as Chairman of the Board of Visitors at Cornell and in a similar capacity for the last 5 years at Yale. The number one problem at these institutions in making rapid moves has been dealing with the teaching hospital.

It is clear from this conference that as leaders in the field, we have to do a better job of educating the public, our trustees, the elected officials at the state level, and federal officials as to what academic health centers are really all about. We need to emphasize that this great national resource needs to be preserved as we enter this era of rapid change.

The Academic Health Center and Health
Care Reform, edited by R. Snyderman,
M.C. Rogers, and V.Y. Saito.
Raven Press, Ltd., New York © 1995.

We Must Stand for Quality

Roscoe R. Robinson, M.D.

Obviously, the future of academic health centers is surrounded by considerable uncertainty and some anxiety as we worry about the impact of health care reform. It appears that our institutions are potentially vulnerable to reform, for reasons that all of you understand.

One of the code words for that is "managed care," because we are relatively high in cost, because we tend to be specialty-oriented, and because we have a limited primary-care base.

A number of strategies have been identified, most of which fall into the rubric of development of a vertically integrated health care system, a network, distributed primary care base, or whatever terms you wish to use.

Some possibilities are a primary care clinic without walls, primary care IPAs, purchaser practices, directly operated primary care clinics, or a combination of all of the above with or without an MSO.

The academic health centers with which I am familiar have not yet made definitive choices. They have not yet selected the processes that are going to be necessary under reform, much less figured out how to position themselves for entry into this new environment coming our way like a freight train.

Cosmetic changes are not going to carry the day. Nevertheless, I believe that adaptation to the new environment will be evolutionary. It will not occur overnight, and much cultural change is going to be required.

There was great concern about funding expressed yesterday in terms of the importance of public or legislative understanding and recognition. The understanding of the interdependence of our revenue streams and the degree to which cross-subsidization occurs among our principal missions is important. Never, at least in my working life, have all of our funding streams been so threatened simultaneously.

We have always had one crisis or another. New crises include the patient care funding stream, professional fees, and direct and indirect costs of research and training. One might even include the cap on tax-free debt, at least if one is a representative of a private university. It is clear that we need better data on the amount of cross-subsidization among our missions as well as the amount of subsidy, per se, for medical education, graduate medical education, and research.

It is good that the current administration has recognized the special costs of academic health centers, because it may be impossible, or at least very difficult for some of us to compete on price alone. It will be to some degree, price–price–price, which means that cost containment is an absolute must.

As we work to influence government at the state and federal levels, we have to remember that our institutions and the markets in which they exist are heterogeneous. What may be good for one is not necessarily good for another. An approach to networking may be better for one institution than another. All of us will have to understand our true costs much better than ever before, including the cost of education at all levels.

Such changes are going to be required, irrespective of the outcome of the federal debate, because, at least in our market, these changes are coming at us full steam on the private initiative alone. We are going to have to justify our value, and that means investment and information systems, and some subsidy may well be needed.

We will have to consider new missions. That may mean changing our curriculum to produce better generalists than we currently produce and changing the behavior of our citizenry and our marketplaces.

Investor-owned companies in our market are entering and buying covered lives. Access to capital will be a problem for all of us. Some may wish to look cautiously at relationships with investor-owned companies.

The fundamental remaining question for all of us is: What should we do and how should we do it? One must remain committed to values we hold high. We must protect our missions in research and education as best we can.

Will we fail if we succeed? That is an important consideration we need to be aware of at all times. All of us need to adopt a strategy that includes access to covered lives and control of management of the premium. The priorities are there. That means operation of a managed care plan.

It is important not to take on more than we can manage. We are the innovators and the builders, and we are the Keepers of the Flame. We must stand for quality in all that we do. All of us have yet to recognize the great latent power inherent in these institutions which will be mobilized when that cultural change is effected. Management of the clash of two cultures is one of our greatest challenges, and managing that clash has to occur.

If we depend on government for our survival, we must accept the political risk of the vicissitudes of government. We can remain private, or we can try for a combination of both. I prefer the latter course.

The Academic Health Center and Health Care Reform, edited by R. Snyderman, M.C. Rogers, and V.Y. Saito. Raven Press, Ltd., New York © 1995.

Government Control or Market Control?

J. Alexander McMahon, J.D.

There is another side. Before you take that easy road, you ought to explore it very carefully. If you remove the health system, the educational system, or any system from the regular part of the economy, then you have to put it in the hands of the government. The leaders of the government come out of the same entrepreneurial side that you want to get away from. If you think they will deal with you gently, I would beg to disagree. They will be worse than the entrepreneurs themselves.

I want to end on a note of optimism. Academic health centers have dealt with change before, and they can again. The United States cannot exist without the roles that the academic health centers play.

The issue is how we want to deal with the future. Do you want to shape it or do you want to let it shape you?

I have five brief observations. First, change is coming. Do not be preoccupied totally with Washington or the State Capitols. Business is a far more important player than that "sleeping giant" that I tried to awaken down here 25 years ago when I was with Blue Cross and Blue Shield. I could never stir the "sleeping giant" then. Now, it is awake, and it probably understands this system better than some of you do.

Business people, the employer, the buyer of health coverage, know that costs cannot be constrained externally. We have tried it on the government side with Certificate of Need and Rate Review. We tried it on the private side with managed care, preadmission certification, and other strategies, and they do not work. Doctors and hospitals beat it every time.

Employers know that costs can be constrained by changing the provider incentives, as capitation does with all the providers living within a fixed preset amount. It is better fixed by negotiation between the providers and the payers, including the enrollees who will have a stake in it themselves, rather than a budget set by government.

If I am correct, then medical education must change to reflect the post-education professional life of physicians. I do not believe you can educate students only to take care of sick people if their professional lives are going to be devoted to taking care of an enrolled population and trying to deal with health.

Please give up the single-payer option and the government assurance of the future of the academic health center. It would mean a huge shift in the dollar flow. It would mean large new taxes. It would mean great government interference. It is not the American way of doing things, and I do not believe business will buy it, especially since they have come to some understanding of this system and do not like government anyway.

I would urge you to support a system in which the individual can exercise an option, not for an individual provider, not at the point of service, but a choice of systems.

Then cost will not be the only issue, because image and the perception of quality will come into play. The individual can make a choice with his wallet, and he or she is likely to choose both perceived quality and actual quality. Some will choose fee-for-service, as well as a capitated plan. You need to be ready to play in that market.

Academic health centers need to learn more about living under capitation and about insurance and the risks that it covers. For example, most employers with 1,000 or more employees do not have health insurance in the true sense. They use an insurance company for enrollment and claims paying, not to insure the risk. They are at risk themselves, and they understand it. That is the reason they are beginning to awaken.

Academic centers need to learn more about money, like how to get it, how to use it, and what substitutes for it. You do not necessarily have to buy a practice; you can contract with some of these practices with the dollars flowing out in the future.

You must decide whether you want government control with all that implies and the difficulty of recovering from governmental error, or marketplace control and the allocation of resources where it is much easier to change directions if mistakes are made.

Some of you think you are approaching a fork in the road. One fork says tragedy and the other says catastrophe and you are faced with choosing wisely. I believe you have come to a fork in the road, and I urge you to take it.

The Academic Health Center and Health Care Reform, edited by R. Snyderman, M.C. Rogers, and V.Y. Saito. Raven Press, Ltd., New York © 1995.

General Discussion

Dr. Rabkin: I have a question for Bill Kelley. In determining the number of specialists, was that based on what the department of neurosurgery felt it needed, or was it a projection of future national needs and the resulting diminution in the number of neurosurgeons who were going to be trained, according to some scheme in the future?

Dr. Kelley: The question that I posed to each of the chairmen was, "What will it take for you to continue to have one of the top five academic training programs in the country in your discipline?"

I assumed that if we are training any subspecialists in the future, we ought to be doing our share at the University of Pennsylvania. Our institution ought to be competitive and to be training subspecialists as well as generalists.

The RRC requirements are quite clear for the specialties and subspecialties, particularly for the surgical disciplines. It is relatively easy to see what you need to have in terms of flow of patients to meet those requirements.

It is also clear that if you want to have one of the top academic training programs, you have to have a substantial breadth of accredited subspecialties.

Orthopaedic surgery is an example. To have one of the top training programs in orthopaedic surgery, you need a foot and ankle doctor, a hand doctor, a spine doctor, and a sports medicine doctor. Not only that, you cannot just have one of them, you have to have two or three, because they like to talk to each other.

The key was that I asked them to look at this from a training perspective in terms of the kind of patients they needed for their training program, not the kind of revenue they needed to support their mission.

Whatever happens, there will be some training left for every subspecialty. It is our responsibility as a leading institution to provide that training and to be competitive for whatever mechanism is selected to provide that training.

Dr. Rogers: One of the calculations Dr. Kelley explained was that there were hundreds of full-time faculty and a different calculation for the total number of faculty.

Dr. Kelley: 275 and 610.

Dr. Rogers: What happens if we have 610 checks to cut and only enough clinical work for 275 people?

Dr. Kelley: In essence, in institutions like ours, everyone has to pay his own way by the work he or she performs. As you know, the major missing piece is who is going to pay for education.

The era is coming to an end when it will be possible for physicians to generate enough clinical revenue from 30% to 50% of their time to take care of their whole salary plus some extra for the institution. However they allocate their time, they will have to generate the support for it, whether it be research or patient care. There will be no way that they can support their education time, and this is one of our most serious problems. How will education be paid for when we lose our ability to cost shift?

Dr. Rogers: I wanted to raise that issue because everyone talks about downsizing the hospitals as if the hospital is a pile of bricks. It is really the practice locus for the vast majority of the faculty.

Then we do another calculation in which we have enough clinical income to pay about a third of that. We have to discuss how we are going to deal with the faculty implications.

The word "excellence" comes through the definition of faculty. You are defining excellence as having all these orthopaedic surgeons who specialize in a specific joint. That is one definition of excellence from the training point of view.

The financial base, the clinical practice base, the hospital base, and the educational base are out of whack. They are no longer in the same diagram. They are starting to dissemble, and somewhere we have to be able to put them back together.

Dr. Relman: Many problems affect us together. For example, how are we going to distribute training opportunities? Who is going to train the neurosurgeons that we need or the orthopaedic surgeons? Will we allow for Darwinian competition, the race going to the swiftest and the smartest, or will we try to plan together? Do we collectively solve any of these problems, or do we have a marketplace that allows everybody to compete as best they can and let the slower ones fall by the wayside?

The American instinct and tradition is to allow the marketplace do it. Is the marketplace really the best way to deal with problems like these, or does the marketplace work well only in certain areas of American life?

For the first time, Americans may have to decide that they have to act collectively to take responsibility for social problems. Medical education is a social problem, not a marketplace problem, just as medical care is a social problem.

We had better keep our minds open to the probability that the marketplace is not going to solve the problem of good medical care and good medical education, just as it cannot solve the problem of medical research.

Dr. New: This is truly a two-culture problem: the academic professional culture and the business culture. They are different but they are moral equivalents. Neither is closer to godliness. Business is no more Philistine and soulless than a high-income physician or a contingent-fee lawyer.

Profit is not bad. Retained service, another more socially acceptable name for profit, is not bad. We have to create what I call profit-power social engines, engines of social betterment that drive themselves on profit, not taxes, not charity, not philanthropy. They drive themselves by delivering value higher than the cost of producing that value.

It is pretty obvious—Darwin was right—any system which spends more on creating value than it gets in return dies. The output has to be more than the input.

We are facing the problem of value system translation. We are merging two cultures, and we are creating a derivative culture that is not the traditional business culture that is our mental model of business. We are creating a different form of business, and we are creating a different form of medicine. This is what the 21st century will be about.

The problem with white male establishment people, the problem with the power structure, the problem with all of us is that we see the future as the length and shadow of our pasts, because it is the past in which we have been quintessentially successful. We are the successful products of that system. Therefore, we believe that the future should repeat the past. It does not work that way.

The future will go to the fastest, it will go to the swiftest, it will go to brightest, it will go to the best capitalized, but it will go. We have to be up in the engines, not back in the caboose.

Dr. Petersdorf: The worst way you can plan for the number and size of specialties is to ask the chairmen of your specialty departments for their estimates. They all think their specialty programs are among the top five. There are 126 medical schools in the AAMC, and 126 of them think they represent the top five.

The critical-mass concept is wistful in today's era. I understand why you need to have a shoulder surgeon and a knee surgeon, but one orthopedic surgeon ought to suffice. If the people in Philadelphia want to talk to one another, you do not need two or three of one specialty at the University of Pennsylvania. Let the knee surgery expert at the University of Pennsylvania talk to the knee surgery expert at Temple University.

That is a somewhat cynical way of saying that our manpower planning has to be collective. It is no longer possible for each program to be autonomous, not if we want training programs to be smaller, more compact, and more efficient. Somehow small is in violation of our academic values. You hear it from your faculty all the time. You hear it from your chairmen. I maintain that culture has to change.

Dr. Sloan: We, in this room, will have no control over whether there is a market solution, and this discussion is a diversion of energy. There will be a marketplace, and there will have to be competition. The organizations represented here will have to compete.

There is an opportunity to influence GME and GME financing, and that is budget-social responsibility as is the research activities of the institution. That is a public function and deserves some concentrated effort.

Capital flows to efficient producers to produce what the market wants. Those who do produce will have capital. It may be accumulated capital from the past, but the future hinges on that.

The question was raised, Should we be insurers? It is possible that we should.

Basic to this is reducing costs, producing a quality product on a unit basis, good low per diems, outpatient care that is both good quality, and low-unit service.

The next question is, How well can care be managed? Do we have a comparative advantage in taking these patients in and turning them out with a quality product at low cost?

Finally, we come to the insurance functions. Insurers involve people who bear risk. They manage claims, and they prevent losses.

We probably have some comparative advantage on loss prevention since that represents utilization review, and physicians can do that very well. I would doubt whether we have a comparative advantage of risk bearing.

Dr. Mulvihill: I have a copy of an interesting article from the *Harvard Magazine* of January/February 1994 called, "The Medical/Industrial Complex" about the creation of Harvard Science Partners, Inc. I am sure this partnership was built with a lot of controversy. Some people carefully seeking to try to preserve the values and the welfare and the reputation of the university, have tried to put a structure together to deal with problems of reduced flow of money to research and capitalize more on using the intellectual capital of the university to help the research effort.

They have gone from $500,000 when it was founded in 1988 to $3.6 million this year, and they are making arrangements with private corporations and providing incentives for faculty and others within the context of the values of the university. Maybe this is the approach we should take as we try to reconcile the two cultures in the arena of health services.

Mr. Lane: I represent the business end of Kaiser Permanente, and I believe we share almost all of the values of our Permanente partners. We are having the same sort of problems because we have a successful past and are now struggling to deal with them.

Nonprofit organizations need capital, too. Last year we generated $1.3 billion in capital. We have many uses for that money, and we want to continue to generate it.

Capital is not free. Do not be deluded that big insurance companies have deep pockets and that they will give you money for nothing. They will not do that. Capital carries a price.

If you want to use excess profits to fund something like education and research, this will happen after you have met all your capital requirements. The only place you can get excess is out of improved efficiencies or premium pricing.

You have either got to do better on the efficiency standard, or somebody has to believe you are better at quality and pay more for your services than they would pay somebody else.

We believe that education and research are public goods and should be paid for with public funds. We strongly support those provisions in the Clinton bill.

We are a little concerned about the amount, but more concerned that the provision in the bill remain that says that all payers, including the self-insured, will be charged the surcharge so we can equalize the playing field and support necessary education and research.

Many of us think that there will be less money available than there is now. That will happen when you put all that money in the pool, and the excess capacity starts becoming more evident to politicians.

Dr. Kelley: In the final analysis, the move that we are witnessing now will do a great deal to improve the quality and the value of health care. I am excited about the opportunity to build a patient care network involving a large number of patients for whom we can take responsibility.

Putting in the information systems, the quality-improvement systems, and all the systems one can implement to make sure that we are providing the highest quality care at the lowest possible cost will be positive changes. The patient will ultimately be the beneficiary of these changes. I am looking forward to being a participant in that.

As we begin to develop our thinking about how best to practice superb preventive medicine, to implement the kinds of genetic counseling and diagnostic techniques that will be available, and to try to implement procedures that are in the patient's best interest, one concern I have is that we could make a very big investment up front in our patient population, but if that population is mobile, we could lose our shirts.

Consider that the breast cancer gene comes along or the colon cancer gene, and we put in a system to be able to detect who has that gene and then to provide appropriate services. That could be very expensive.

On the other hand, if that patient population is so mobile that you experience a shift of hundreds of thousands of patients to another HMO, the net effect will be that we really will not be able to implement the care we desire. How does one protect against that?

Professor Reinhardt: This morning you had fresh milk, and you never wondered how it got here. It did not get here because of anything but a lot of people pursuing profits. The market provides most things that we human beings want, and the force of that should never be underestimated.

You can conceive of it as two circles that overlap. There are some things a market-driven system cannot accomplish. Today's *New York Times* has a front-page story on the plight of American children, stating that there are many children who do not get decent medical care.

In a way, that is a product of a market system. You cannot blame a particular player in the market, but markets do not serve where there is no purchasing power, even if we have values that say they should.

Therefore, economists in their teaching always identified what we call merit wants. I want our children to have X, Y, and Z and there is no purchasing power. Somehow, I have to get it there. Usually, economists prefer to put vouchers into the hands of these children or their parents, and then have competition, rather than giving institutions money and let it drain down in a paternalistic manner.

That is our bias. We may be wrong, but we do not trust institutional grants much, because, while markets are not very good at serving needs that have value where there is no purchasing power, I believe it is also fair to say that nonprofit institutions and governments are not very good at downsizing. They are not very good at cutting out waste, which really upsets an economist. One of the values of a for-profit business enterprise is not to waste society's resources. That is not usually a value that drives nonprofit institutions or the government.

Instead of criticizing each other, we should recognize each other's weaknesses and strengths. There is some overlap where academic health centers are just as competitive, just as tough, and serve just as well as a for-profit company would.

You have to tell your story better. Markets cannot fund treating the poor, research, and teaching very well. You have to put before the public and the Congress the credible stories of what you would need in the way of support.

The problem in the past with the health system is there has been too much "crying wolf," and that's a dangerous thing to do as we go forward. If you have a crisis that needs addressing, you have to be really sure that it is a crisis and back it up with numbers. I think that can be done. Go forward in this market and multiply!